Your Inner River of Peace

Ten Messages of Love

Candace Jean Newman

Your Inner River of Peace
Ten Messages of Love

Copyright © 2020 by Candace Jean Newman and
Touch With Oils® Institute LLC
Eustis, FL
All rights reserved.

No part of this work may be used or reproduced, transmitted, stored or used in any form or by any means graphic, electronic, or mechanical, including but not limited to photocopying, recording, scanning, digitizing, tapping, Web distribution, information networks or information storage and retrieval systems, or in any manner whatsoever without the prior written permission of the publisher, except in the case of brief quotations embodied in critical reviews and certain other noncommercial uses permitted by copyright law. For permission requests, contact "Attention: Permissions Coordinator", at info@TouchWithOilsInstitute.com

ISBN: 978-1-7332824-0-6 (color version)
ISBN: 978-1-7332824-2-0 (black and white version)
eBook ISBN 978-1-7332824-1-3
Printed in the United States

This book is not intended as a substitute for the medical advice of physicians. The reader should regularly consult a physician in matters relating to his/her health and particularly with respect to any symptoms that may require diagnosis or medical attention.

TOUCH WITH OILS® AND THE OIL LADY® ARE REGISTERED TRADEMARKS.
ALL RIGHTS RESERVED.

Dedication

The experience of writing this book and all it encompasses has been done in honor of my loving Mom and Dad, Elizabeth June Wagner Tooker and William Riecks Tooker. Mom always encouraged me to paint, and Dad always encouraged me to write. I am finally following my heart doing two things I love, reminding me of the two extraordinary people who gave me life.

These writings are dedicated to you for all you have been, all you are, and all you will become from this day forward.

There is a place in our hearts that yearns for our connection to our Inner River of Peace. This yearning often feels like a struggle.

However, the knowing that *your* Inner River of Peace exists and the action of showing up and holding the vision to connect to it, make the heart happy. This knowing can turn into a joyful thing. The purpose of the book is to offer *Ten Messages of Love*, ushering in the Inner River of Peace that flows through our hearts.

> Love starts in the heart
> The place where God always is…
> Patiently waiting for us,
> To quietly, come home.
>
> Candace Jean Newman

May you come home to your heart again and again, with each of The Messenger's *Ten Messages of Love*.

With all of my heart, I thank you for being here.

Your Inner River of Peace: Ten Messages of Love

CONTENTS

Dedication iii
Letter from the Author 1
Who is The Messenger? 13
Ways to Enjoy This Book 21

MESSAGE ONE
Show Up and Hold the Vision **35**
    My Personal Story *36*
    Interpretation *40*
    Ideas and Actions *51*
    Contemplative Moments *54*

MESSAGE TWO
Look at the Sky **57**
    My Personal Story *58*
    Interpretation *64*
    Ideas and Actions *73*
    Contemplative Moments *77*

MESSAGE THREE
Focus on the Light and Love **81**
    My Personal Story *82*
    Interpretation *87*
    Ideas and Actions *93*
    Contemplative Moments *97*

REVIEW MESSAGES 1-3 .... **101**

MESSAGE FOUR
Anchor Way Down Deep **107**
    My Personal Story *109*
    Interpretation *113*
    Ideas and Actions *120*
    Contemplative Moments *124*

MESSAGE FIVE
Keep Me with You **129**
    My Personal Story *131*
    Interpretation *134*
    Ideas and Actions *138*
    Contemplative Moments *142*

Table of Contents

MESSAGE SIX
Don't Resist the Web of Life **145**
    My Personal Story 146
    Interpretation 156
    Ideas and Actions 158
    Contemplative Moments 162

REVIEW MESSAGES 4-6 .... **167**

MESSAGE SEVEN
The Power Out Here **173**
    My Personal Story 174
    Interpretation 180
    Ideas and Actions 185
    Contemplative Moments 188

MESSAGE EIGHT
Trust Me Like Never Before **193**
    My Personal Story 194
    Interpretation 202
    Ideas and Actions 208
    Contemplative Moments 212

MESSAGE NINE
The Coal and The Diamond **217**
    My Personal Story 219
    Interpretation 223
    Ideas and Actions 228
    Contemplative Moments 233

REVIEW MESSAGES 7-9 .... **237**

MESSAGE TEN
You Are Called **245**
    My Personal Story 247
    Interpretation 254
    Ideas and Actions 260
    Contemplative Moments 264

REVIEW MESSAGES 1-10 .... **269**

The Power of the 5 Senses Plus 2 279
Essential Oils as Soulful Elements 329
Build Your Own Home of Cards 369
What Happened Here? 375
Conclusion 381
Acknowledgements 387
About the Author 389

Letter from the Author

There are often things that come along in life that seem to be saving our life. These are things that really nurture and sustain us. *Your Inner River of Peace* is an invitation to explore and discover the golden nuggets of wisdom and love each Message has for you. The Messages take you deeper into this reservoir of peace that lives in the heart and soothes the soul. A bit of joy lives here too.

The research for this book has been the seventy years of living in the laboratory of my life so far. My travels, from the top of Huayna Picchu to the deserts of Saudi Arabia, have shown we all experience our share of struggles and thrills. The deep frustration of our self-doubts and fears can lead us to new insights of who we truly are. In the midst of it all, we find courage, compassion, and even inspiration. We can claim resilience and regeneration as we strengthen our stance in our Inner River of Peace.

In addition to the truly wonderful and loving people in my life, starting with my mother and father, I am so grateful for the other world of existence that periodically seems to save my life. It keeps showing me what I need to know when it believes I need to know it. This happens in its own time frame and usually not the minute I think I need and want it.

The first of these otherworld experiences are The Messages that come in on a wave of peace with a pause of stillness. They were delivered from seemingly nowhere at the least expected moments. Then, there are certainly times I wonder if I lost my connection to them. I know better by now. It is my own challenge. The wisdom and love show up when the time is right.

Once The Messages come in, they are an anchor in my life going forward. As time marches on, The Messages reveal more wisdom for different situations. These Messages are universal truths delivering their wisdom relative to each life situation in space and time. Sometimes it's a hint or insight of something in the future. I always knew these Messages were not just for me.

Letter From The Author

The second of the otherworld experiences are the essential oils and their unlimited potential on many levels. They initially showed up in 1989, when I was actively searching for help to resolve health issues. I had been to fifteen doctors and had several surgeries over six years. I was desperately seeking relief from physical pain and emotional exhaustion. The love, the instant knowing, and the affinity I felt for essential oils brought tears to my eyes. I realized this was not just about my health. They were to be part of my life's purpose and came in to be my next profession.

The third element that reveals wisdom and love while nurturing and sustaining me is Mother Nature. She gives us her joy and healing balms through all her seasons, elements, beauty, and rhythms. The sights and the colors, the sounds and the silence, the breeze and the stillness are all part of her majestic glory. Nature is a place many people go to feel the presence of God. Our Inner River of Peace is here.

All of these things from the nonphysical and physical world are soulful elements. We recognize this kind of love that comes from both sides of creation and existence because it touches us on a very deep level. It leads us to pause, gives us the chills, and makes us feel at home with our heart and soul.

This book brings together ten of The Messages of Love received throughout my life. Each Message is accompanied with a personal story of my life's situation that brought in The Message. The wisdom plays out in many ways.

I present a chapter on *The Power of the 5 Senses Plus 2,* to provide you with options to use with The Messages. Using our senses with The Message enhances the experience. The synergy moves the experience from the intellectual level to our cellular behavior. Our spirit can soar.

Essential oils are powerful elements from the earth and have the ability to amplify The Message's wisdom and enrich the meaning on a spiritual and cellular level. This is due to the physiology of our unique nose-brain connection. I had not heard of essential oils when The Messages started coming to me, and I have always been oversensitive to smells. I only present them here because, after thirty years of experiencing them with clients and customers, I see how they enrich people's lives. They assist us through transitions of all kinds on an expansive level. I invite you to explore the royal mission essential oils have with us in my chapter: *Essential Oils as Soulful Elements.*

We can't give away what we don't have within us, so it all starts with us. These Messages, along with simple techniques and newly created *holy habits*, serve to strengthen our personal relationship with our Inner River of Peace. Then we can be more of our stellar self of heroic proportions. As long as we are alive, this

Letter From The Author

is part of a worthwhile purpose for being here. We become part of the light of life. We become more of who we really are. This process gives us glimpses of our true talents, purpose, and the omnipresent kind of love.

Our Inner River of Peace holds everything we need to navigate the rapids, waterfalls, stagnant eddies, and the rocks of life. Instead of anger, resentment, fear, and all kinds of negative dross, we can anchor way down deep in compassion and strength. The Messages help us and guide us home to our heart's inner sanctum. Remember, all things are possible. Life is a journey of great courage.

> *Courage is being scared to death*
> *and saddling up anyway.*
> John Wayne

I've always said it takes courage on a daily basis to live our lives. I keep saddling up the best I know how. After all, what's the alternative?

Each chapter of a Universal Message of Love serves us all as an unlimited source of guidance, courage, and faith. There are different perspectives of wisdom at different times in our lives. So, let's saddle up together and embrace each season at it comes.

Your Inner River of Peace is an unlimited source of love and compassion. The very substance of rivers being water naturally nurtures us. We were formed and born in water. Our bodies are made of approximately 70% water. Water is the liquid gold of life. It glistens and dances with the sun. No wonder we love getting in water. We become weightless and free of aches and pains, physically and mentally.

We all have times of rapids and waterfalls in our lives. We also know there are times of calm waters. Seasons change, and these Messages from The Messenger are life preservers to weather the storms and keep our head above water. Put on your life preserver and honor the wisdom that is yours in each message.

Life is not easy. There were times when I felt like I was in the desert with no oasis in sight. The river was dry, and I questioned my ability to carry on. Does this sound familiar to you? These times are scary and are often accompanied by exhaustion and health challenges. Two of these especially potent experiences in my life come to mind.

The first was after my father passed away in 2000. I spent a month by myself with an Inca Yachak (shaman) and two of his Inca apprentices high up in the Andes of Ecuador above the cloud line. The wooden cabin had no electricity, and ice-cold water came in through a pipe from a mountain stream above us. We cooked over a wood fire in the middle of the floor and slept with bed bugs chewing on us at night. The shaman suggested I stay there alone. I agreed, and I was left there for four days and three nights. It was

Letter From The Author

certainly a test on many levels and dimensions. As it got late on the fourth day, I didn't know if anyone was ever going to come back. The water pipe went dry. I was starting to think of additional survival tools. What if they fell off the mountain and no one knows I'm here? There was no walking out to anything. My fear turned to courage as I anchored deep and made a plan. By the grace of God, the shaman came back later that evening with the two apprentices.

> *Anchor way down deep*
> *in the bottom of the ocean,*
> *and ride the waves.*
> *Everything is OK.*
>
> *Message Four*

The second time was when my first husband and I crashed, burned, and went broke with a twelve-court tennis club we owned. We made the club successful in every way, except financially for us. We worked ourselves to the bone and averaged about three hours of sleep a night for about thirteen months. Too many big money issues came up. Our pockets were not deep enough to sustain unanticipated challenges, like sinkholes in the parking lot. In the process, we also lost our home and needed to sell our four rental properties at losses. After moving back to Naples, Florida, we lived out of suitcases while renting a home and bartering tennis lessons. I was up in the middle of many nights wondering if this would ever end and how we were going to get out of it. The chest pains and exhaustion didn't help. Eventually, the rapids cleared, and we got back on our feet again.

Keep Me with You,
just Keep Me with You.

Message Five

Each time The Messages connect me to my Inner River of Peace. This is their mission. There is a strange sense that everything, no matter what the outcome, is going to be okay—somehow.

The Messages have their own timing. I have gotten better at learning to trust them. They are ushered in on a wave of peace. There is a pause, a lovely stillness, a moment in time. It's always the wisdom I need. Sometimes, I don't realize this until later. If we wait for divine timing, we usually don't have to go back and fix a knee-jerk decision. Patience with a big dose of faith and trust is the way to go. Not easy for us. However, the rewards are worth it.

Wherever our thoughts and emotions go, there goes our body.

Yes, there are rapids of drama in life—and we can get through them.

Yes, there are eddies of stagnant green goop—and we can get out of them.

Yes, there are rocks and riverbanks banging us up—and we can survive this too.

Letter From The Author

Writing this book has been a very personal soul call for me. It has taken me back to reading my journals for the first time since they were written. It serves as a bit of an autobiography, as I relived and wrote each personal story. Each Message has taken me deeper into its meaning on a broader scale. Now, these Messages are even dearer, as I share them with the world.

Getting into *your* Inner River of Peace is one of the most exciting adventure trips of a lifetime. Each step is part of our own personal river-road map. We get better at honoring and supporting all the parts of us that are often scattered. Our spirit no longer needs to be broken or disconnected from the rest of us. Marrying our heart and mind with our soul and spirit can be our greatest love affair. How do we create this?

> *A jug fills drop by drop.*
> Buddha

We do this one Message at a time. Message One is: *Show Up and Hold the Vision.* You are already doing this. You have already started the process because you are here with your precious heart. You have entered the *Circle of Compassion in Action* The Messages create through the geometric symbols.

May The Messages serve you with golden nuggets throughout your life even better than they have served me. Explore, experience, and be inspired.

Rarely do we read a book in which 100% of it rings true for us. Stay with me panning for your golden nuggets and find the ones that assist you. If you find even one golden nugget for your life right now, then my dream has been realized. The Messages relate to each situation in a pointed and highly personal way. This is part of the beauty, the grace, and the blessing of our life adventures.

I offer you a respite from the busyness of life, from the hurried rush of the masses, and from the noise of complexity. Allow each Message to come to the rescue. I hold the belief, vision, and prayer that The Messages continue to serve you throughout your life with expanded perspective, understanding, and compassion for yourself and others. They continue to do this for me. God willing, and the creek don't rise, I will continue to receive them and be full of thanksgiving every step of the way.

Be ready and excited to accept, honor, and trust who you are and who you are becoming. Embrace the heart of the explorer within. My life experiences of pain and joy have taught me to keep asking for guidance, keep seeking the courage to follow it, and keep knocking on the door of faith. May *your* Inner River of Peace be with you. It will become one of your best friends.

I love the Inner River of Peace in all of us. After we acknowledge and embrace it in ourselves, we are able to see it in others. Our Rivers of Peace flow into the big ocean of universal existence.

The river of life continues whether we are going with the current, struggling up stream, stuck in the eddy, smashed against the side, tossed around by the rapids, falling over the waterfall—or flowing peacefully at one of those "Praise God" moments when all is well in our world. Rain or shine the Inner River of Peace exists. It helps us be resilient in this world of continual activity.

When we are in the rapids and tumbling over rocks, we don't know which way is up. We lose our compass and sense of direction. It seems like an impossible situation. Caregivers know this all too well. Anchor deep and grab one of these Messages of Love. Muster up your courage and keep going. A certain kind of love comes to the rescue.

Gather these golden nuggets glittering with light and love. To lighten the load at times, hum a favorite song like the one I love below. When I hum or sing this on my walks, my step instantly picks up. Then repeat *your* Inner River of Peace Message or put it to a favorite tune and sing away!

> *Row, row, row your boat* (not someone else's)
> *Gently down the stream* (not up the stream)
> *Merrily, Merrily, Merrily, Merrily* (struggle-free)
> *Life is but a dream.* (don't give up on your dream)

Whatever you do, hang on to your dreams. Don't throw them overboard. It took until age seventy to get my dream book written.

Two of my go-to themes in my life, flow through this book:
Stop, Look, and Listen (SLL)

Slow, Still, and Simple (SSS)

Then I remember to be full of thanks. Life is better if we treat each day with the art of giving thanks the best we can.

I am delighted, as your river guide, to have you on this trip with me. My heart smiles thinking about the wisdom and peace waiting for you. Continue to love, honor, and support who you are around every bend in the river. In doing and being this, we can honor others. We remember to hold a reverence for life in all things great and small. A grace beyond words.

In reality you are *your* Inner River of Peace. These Messages are here to reveal more of the wonderful self of you.

Love is the question
the answer
the lock
and the key.

It all starts with us being anchored in our Inner River of Peace with *Ten Messages of Love.*

Love,

Candace Jean Newman

Who is The Messenger?

What it is that dwelleth here I know not,
but my heart is full of awe
and tears trickle down.
Japanese 11th C.

Have you ever felt a Power much greater than you come in and sort something out for you? Perhaps it delivered a message at the perfect time or protected you from a situation. Throughout my life, part of this Power greater than us has been a Voice delivering a Message on a wave of peace. It is always accompanied by a pause of stillness. After seventy years, I am still full of awe and tears still trickle down.

The Messenger, who is delivering The Message, is personal to each of us. The spirit of The Messenger gives us the wisdom and the might that we need at that moment. It is an inexhaustible reservoir of our Inner River of Peace.

Not by might, nor by power, but my spirit.
Zachariah 4:6

I was brought up in Chevy Chase, Maryland, and my family went to a lovely Methodist church made of stone, with wooden pews, cathedral ceilings, and beautiful stained-glass windows. One Sunday when I was quite young, my parents asked me if I wanted to go to Sunday school or church. I immediately chose church. Sunday school was too much talking. As I sat in church that Sunday, I vividly remember a certain experience, and I revisit this in my heart-mind often.

This particular Sunday morning, I was sitting in a wooden pew with my little legs sticking straight out. I was looking high up on my left at the beautiful light dancing through the large stained-glass windows. I glanced up at Minister Richmond, a lovely tall grey-haired man, speaking from the pulpit. I looked around at everyone intently focused on him. He was the type of minister with the kind, calm, assertive voice everyone loved. I remember thinking to myself: *I wonder why everyone is listening to him, when they could be sitting here listening to God.* Of course, it would be good to do both; however, my childlike mind of wonder was at work (or play). This, along with the serenity of the organ, was my experience of going to church. I still cherish this sense of childlike awe and wonder. We must not let the ways of the world take this sense of wonder away from us.

Thus, The Messenger for me is God.

I don't recall The Messages with their peace and stillness before that experience. It was around age seven. That's also around the time I was in Children's Hospital in Washington DC, in and out of consciousness with a high fever caused by mumps, encephalitis, and an inflamed pancreas. The timing was interesting—a coincidence or a life event?

I do know this connection is deeply comforting and The Messages of Love are here for all of us. They serve and guide us through life and remind us peace and stillness are possible. Sometimes, we only get a little glimpse, and that is enough for which to be grateful and to know it's there. There is peace in the knowing.

Nature has always been one of my places where I sense the wonder of God. Nature is a place of wisdom and beauty. If we create the time and space to show up and be still, it also becomes a valued place of introspection. God can speak to us here through this marvelous creation of innate intelligence. Rivers, mountains, trees, and flowers; as well as the sky, the ocean, and the animals are all part of the soulful elements of existence. Since we are a most exquisite soulful element ourselves, we sense this affinity, a remembrance and a beauty all of its own. Our soul instantaneously recognizes other soulful elements that cross our path. Our hearts feel at home. There is a sense of grace and ease here. Sometimes it feels like the ever flowing gentle yet powerful breath of God.

> *God's grandest cathedral is Nature,*
> *in all her Majestic Garb.*

Yes, The Messenger is very personal to each of us. It is the result of our heritage, life experiences, beliefs, and convictions. There is a spirit and a power that is greater than all of us. Reflect on this source. When have you sensed this in your life, and what were you doing?

From your perspective and meaningful life, who is The Messenger to you? For some, it is a Guardian Angel, a saint, or sage, a Higher Power, or a strong sense of the Divine. In Greek and Arabic, the word *Messenger* means *Angel.* Angels send us messages, comfort, protection, and healings. Sometimes there are aromas in the air, such as, roses or oranges. There is a sense of the mysterious with The Messenger, which we learn to cherish and love. We don't need to try and understand it. Accepting it with ease is an act of faith and ultimately trust on a higher level.

> *The most beautiful thing we can experience is the mysterious.*
> *It is the source of all true art and science.*
> Albert Einstein

You will notice that sometimes The Messenger comes in as "we," such as: *We will bring in all that you need.* Other times it comes in as "I" or "me," such as: *You must Trust me like never before, if you want to survive.* I wouldn't pretend to explain the absolute of this ever-fulfilling source. It runs deep in the core of our being. The Messages have a mysterious ability to gently shift us into a most profound sense of well-being. We receive wisdom and peace on a cellular and energetic level, not just intellectually as we read the words.

As we merge with our Inner River of Peace, we can sense this river flows through all of us. Spend some quiet times with The Messenger and set the intent to cultivate this strong loving relationship. You are tapping into *your* Inner River of Peace with each Message. Pan for the golden nuggets that are just for you. They are always there, waiting to be brought to the light.

Just getting a glance and a feeling of this peace now and then, keeps us going. The Messages are universal truths for our heart, spirit, and soul no matter our belief system. They transcend the boundaries within us and between us, as they deliver a peace and serenity that goes beyond our imagination.

Through my travels and experiences with people of all faiths, I have experienced and discovered this Inner River of Peace that runs through all of us. To me, it is God's Love. If we go down deep enough, we can find this endless field of compassion. Finding compassion for our self comes first. Then we are able to observe it in others. Finally, we realize all our Inner Rivers of Peace flow into the same omnipresent ocean of existence.

The Messenger with each Message will find us anywhere. It didn't seem to matter whether I was—with the Inca above the cloud line in the Andes of Ecuador, the Saudi women in Saudi Arabia, the Buddhists in Thailand, the Jesuits priests in the mountains of North Carolina, the Benedictine Monks of St. Leo Abbey, the wife of the candlemaker in Cyprus, or in silent retreat on the Pacific Ocean. There were the times I was walking with my parents into a condo they were buying, driving on a highway, riding on a crowded bus in noisy San Francisco, and at the mysterious tippy top of Huayna Picchu in Peru. The Messenger delivering the Inner River of Peace prevailed. Thank goodness, we are not really lost when we're sure we are.

As we take on the journey of finding peace in ourselves, we have this to share with others. Of course, we get thrown into the rapids and up against the riverbanks of life now and then. Thankfully, the season changes, and we get our head above water and back in the gentle flow. There is a quiet power here. It transcends the world of matter and form. Trust the gentle power of the flow. See my poem: *The Path of Yearning Little Heart,* later on in this book.

Who Is The Messenger?

Life is precious. Anchor deep in the love The Messenger has hidden for you in the vibrational frequency of the words in each Message. Realize we are not alone. We are all connected, and from here, we remember the reverence for life in all things and all God's creatures great and small.

Sometimes life feels like we're stuck in the desert and our well has gone dry. We're thirsty to get back to the oasis before we find ourselves so far out, that it's a crawl to get back! Burning out is often the result. The Messenger brings us back to our Inner River of Peace. Smooth waters await.

The river of life presents plenty of challenges around each bend. Thus, finding our Inner River of Peace in the midst of daily life can seem out of reach. The rough waters are part of this existence of duality. By consciously thinking with the heart and feeling with the mind, we make it to calm waters. This is the heart-mind muscle theme I carry throughout the book. It starts to become a natural reaction. Know every section of the river trip continues to make us who we are. There is a time for all seasons. Seasons change. That's the way it is.

I continue to be grateful in my life that God is in charge on a grander scale and goes before us, around us, above us, and within us to light the way. God has our back, and all the rest of us, too. My job is to *Show Up and Hold the Vision*—and *Focus on the Light and Love* so that is what I will magnify. This is not easy when we are in the rapids, praying and waiting for relief and guidance. Each time I trust the Inner River of Peace connection, it builds my strength to trust more. Part of our life purpose is Trust. Deep trust is also one of our biggest challenges.

> *Trust in the Lord with all thine heart*
> *and lean not unto thine own understanding:*
> *in all thy ways acknowledge him,*
> *and he shall direct thy paths.*
> Proverbs 3:5

Tough events and big challenges happen in our lives. They are course corrections in what Paulo Coelho calls *the Path of Our Personal Legend*. As we trust the truth of The Messenger and the truth within us, our Trust will grow stronger and stronger. Here lives the amazing glory of grace.

> *In quietness and trust shall be your strength.*
> Isaiah 30:15

This is a language that goes beyond words, into the field of pure potentiality. May you be embraced by the Great Holy Comforter that continues to reveal your Self to you.

May The Messenger and The Messages in this book, guide you home to *your* Inner River of Peace. It all starts here. You are on your way.

Ways To Enjoy This Book

This book is about creating some new ways to go through each day with *Ten Messages of Love* connecting you to *your* Inner River of Peace. The experiences reveal wisdom and compassion that is unique to your life. There are two constant themes flowing through the book to lead the way to receive the most from each Message.

Stop, Look, and Listen (SLL)

Slow, Still, and Simple (SSS)

Enjoy these two slogan/mantras many times with The Messages. They are continual go-to tools when we are in doubt, feel stuck, or just need a breath of fresh air. Will somebody please throw us a bone?

Stop – is not a harsh command. It is the strength and wisdom of a gentle pause.

Look – simply means to step aside, disengage, and observe or gaze. Clear the field.

Listen – means getting quiet and seeing the space around the subject. Listen to what is really going on.

Then remember:

Slow – is a deliberate pause and a deep breath. The tai chi walk exemplifies *slow*.

Still – is holding open a window, door, or space for something to happen. Be still like a mountain.

Simple – is elegant. There is power, clarity, and peace in focusing on purpose. The Messages are simple.

Your Inner River of Peace is always deep within you, even when you can't find it anymore. This book is an invitation for you to embark on our expedition whose purpose is to anchor you in *your*

Inner River of Peace. The Messages subtly build into lifelong guides to light our way.

My way to be of assistance is this offering of *Ten Messages of Love* that arrived as messages throughout my life. The Messages come on a wave of peace and leave a quiet stillness of grace. The Messages operate on divine timing. The Messages are always just what is needed to carry us home to our Inner River of Peace.

When you read each Message, go beyond the words and my story. See what is here for you. Each Message contains golden nuggets. Own The Message in your own way that serves who you are right now. You will know it's your way if there is a sense of peace, even if you are being asked to take a big step.

Each of the ten chapters of Messages is composed of four parts: My Personal Story, Interpretation, Ideas and Action, and Contemplative Moments. Then The Messages are grouped together into four Review sections. This provides an easy-to-read pattern bringing the synergy of The Messages together.

Each Message is accompanied by its number and unique place in the individual shapes within the completed geometric color wheel. This serves as The Message Mandala leading us into a stronger relationship with our Inner River of Peace. Simply by reading Message One, you have already become a part of this *Circle of Compassion in Action,* a field we meet in together. It is here where *your* Inner River of Peace thrives. They build our trust and deepen our faith by showing us wisdom and peace are possible.

Some of The Messages may really speak to you; some will be more meaningful at another time. There may be one Message that really changes your life. Each Message has more for us the more we keep it in our heart and on our mind.

The chapter on *The Power of the 5 Senses Plus 2* presents ideas to combine with each Message. Together, they enhance your intuition and entrain The Message's wisdom throughout your whole being. The next chapter: *Essential Oils as Soulful Elements*, presents more ideas and options. Choose a sensory stimulus you love or something new you want to experience. *Holy habits* abound.

Many of us have excelled in the intellectual and reasoning part of our minds, often at the expense of our hearts. Our hearts and minds yearn to be together. Excess of either creates the havoc of being out of sorts. Think of the peace we can feel and the brilliant shining stars the heart and mind can become when they merge in their purpose of serving the other. This is sacred synergy and a worthy ideal.

Throughout the book is the novel idea of thinking with the heart and feeling with the mind. I call this our heart-mind muscle. Muscles and neural pathways strengthen with use. They become more powerful with repetition. One continual gentle drop of water on the ground will eventually make a big impression.

Gather up your curiosity and courage. It's time to discover the hidden treasure in each Message unique to you, as the treasure reveals more of your wonderful self. Imagine yourself following your dream-purpose and believing it is possible. The heart and the mind rejoice.

Creating Your Own *Holy Habits* with Each Message

We have lost the sense of holiness in our daily habits, as the busyness of the world takes over. I love this definition of routine, ritual, and habit.

Ritual is routine infused with mindfulness. It is habit made holy.
Kent Nerburn, *Small Graces*

It his beautiful little book, Kent Nerburn reminds us that our cup of coffee in the morning or our morning routine of reading emails or the news—when done with mindfulness—is a ritual, a habit made holy. Taking a walk and getting a morning dose of nature is a delightful *holy habit*. This is a time to be *Slow, Still, and Simple* (SSS). These *holy habits* are healing games and good medicine to our central nervous system, not to mention our spirit and soul, and all the rest of our many parts.

What do you do first thing in the morning, at times during the day, or when you tuck yourself in at night? Each Message can accompany that time. Find ways that flow with ease to assimilate all the goodness.

One of my many *holy habits:* I awaken in the morning with my glass of warm water and lemon. Then I make my special coffee and go into my studio. Holding my cup of coffee with both hands, I slowly do my tai chi walk. I look forward to this process, along with my quiet time of reading, listening, and/or writing. This includes my heart thinking about my intentions, while my mind focuses on feeling it. This is about inspiration, imagination, and a bunch of Trust. My precious dog is part of this *holy habit*, and I get up earlier just for this time to myself.

Your new *holy habits* are contemplative experiences because you have infused them with mindfulness. Meditation, prayer, and quiet pauses touch other parts of your magnificent self. Getting into this energy with focus and integrity, brings inspirational thoughts and feelings into words and actions. Here we find more of who we are and more of what is really important to us.

The big magical key is finding your way to use each Message. Make it a passionate way, flowing with ease through your daily/nightly doings and beings. This is easy. Just breathe and repeat The Message with your thinking heart and feeling mind.

Ways To Enjoy This Book

How to Use This Book

When I first started writing this book, I thought each Message could be a seven-day reboot of love downloading its wisdom as a gateway to *your* Inner River of Peace. Seven is a number of creation and completion. As the book carried on, I sensed each Message might serve best as a daily, weekly, or monthly guide. More importantly, the choice has to be yours. It must be simple and easy for you to do. Here within lies the treasures. The Messages build on each other, as you can see in the symbol they create.

The longer and more meaningful the time invested, the deeper the energy is created to move the words and their vibrations from the intellectual level to a cellular visceral experience. These new thoughts and feelings create new corresponding brain chemistry that is sent to cell membranes throughout the body. Here the cells are getting new information about how to behave. Then we speak and act in a different way. Thinking and behaving with love and wisdom is truly a blessing of another kind.

The *Ten Messages of Love* and our Inner River of Peace are here to push the boundaries on what we think is possible. The Messenger reveals deeper wisdom, the more we use it throughout our life. In this experience, we find divine timing, divine order, and divine grace. Getting a peek of this keeps us going because now we know it's possible.

The key to mastering anything is to meet yourself wherever you are—and move forward from there.

1. Start with Message One and use it for seven days, a month, or your best way.
2. Choose one of the sensory ideas from *The Power of the 5 Senses Plus 2* to enhance The Message.
3. Look at your daily routines and see what *holy habits* you already have and what new ones you might like to create to accompany The Message.

Viewing a Message three times a day seems to be optimal, such as:

1. Begin each morning anchoring The Message with your cup of coffee or in a time to reflect and listen.
2. Put your mind on The Message at lunch or another time of the day.
3. End the day anchoring The Message again while brushing your teeth and/or looking into your eyes in the mirror. Reflect upon your day.

Example with Message Two: Focus on the Light and Love, and That is what You will magnify. Throughout the day notice the light coming through the window, the trees, and the clouds. Look for it everywhere. Notice the kind

Ways To Enjoy This Book

words people say and kind actions they do. When we acknowledge this, it changes our thoughts, feelings, words, and actions. We also start to see things we didn't notice before.

Here are some simple ideas for times to contemplate The Message: morning coffee and routine times in the bathroom, in a shower or bath, in the car at stop lights, while waiting for the microwave to ding or standing in line at the grocery store. Then there is washing dishes, cooking meals, doing chores of any kind, and rubbing the dog's belly. Put The Message under your pillow, in your pocket, on your phone, or a sticky note on the mirror. Don't forget the freedom of looking at the sky or any part of nature, by gazing out the window, dancing or singing The Message.

Moving the body engages our whole vessel. Exercise automatically increases our breathing rate. As we move and breath with The Message, we serve the goodness in ourselves in many ways. Shifted thoughts and feelings are reflected in our mood and spirit. Be inventive and tap into your wellspring of options.

Stop, Look, and Listen (SLL)

We are not looking for more time to add a new thing into your day. We are looking for simple ways to put your thoughts and feelings on the loving wisdom from The Messenger. Share this process with a loved one if you like. Listen to each other's different golden nuggets of wisdom.

Show up each day with your selected Message and allow it to assist, protect, and guide you. Ask The Messenger each day to show you what you need to know. Sometimes it shows us how to follow our dreams. Insights come in when you need to know them.

Explore the ways that let you know you are connected to *your* Inner River of Peace. I call this creating your very own healing games of good medicine. A Native American definition of *medicine* is *anything that connects you to Great Spirit*. Dr. Andrew Weil stated that the words *medicine* and *meditation* share the same root word. No wonder meditation is all about connecting and healing.

Honor and support all that you are now and imagine all you are becoming. Be full-of-thanks and embrace the brilliant bundle of *you*. Yes, every single little cellular part of you is waiting to be loved.

Oh, the Places You'll Go!
Dr. Seuss

We live in worlds of nonsense and truth, fear and love, noise and quiet. With a foot in each world, we yearn to be anchored in our Inner Rivers of Peace. This is where we bring our scattered parts back together. From here, we can recognize each other's Inner River of Peace and remember to hold a reverence for life.

Life is difficult, and life is beautiful.

Life is a struggle, and life flows.

Life can feel stuck, and life holds *your* Inner River of Peace.

May your experiences with the Ten Messages of Love, love you through your life and remind you to hold onto your dreams. Following dreams has divine timing. May you find *your* Inner River of Peace strengthens your trust, deepens your faith, and reveals your truly magnificent self.

> *There are no extra pieces in the universe.*
> *Everyone is here because he or she has a place to fill,*
> *and every piece must fit itself into the big jigsaw puzzle.*
> Deepak Chopra

Most of all, may you gain an expansive perception of the grandeur of the divine Higher Power, the God particle that is in everyone and everything everywhere.

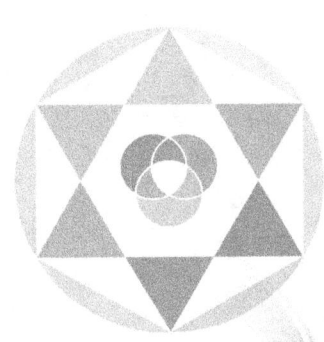

The Messages

Message One
Show Up and Hold the Vision

The Message

*What are you fretting about? Don't you remember?
All YOU agreed to do is:
Show Up and Hold the Vision.
We can do all the rest through you.*

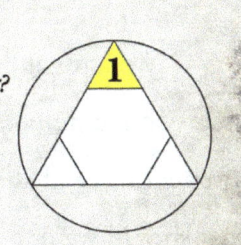

In other words, if we consciously become the open vessel and lay down the armor of struggle and frustration, we will be shown the way. If we don't show up as the vessel, there is nothing through which to work. The power greater than us is ready to help. We simply need to open our tight fists, which reflect our tight mind, and lay down our heavy doubts and worries.

Be still for one breath. Know you are already showing up and holding the vision because you are here right now. Just showing up is a prerequisite to accomplishing something. If we don't show up with our heart and mind open to receive, we're working against ourselves.

My Personal Story

We have all had times when several life events happen all at once. We are desperately trying to think it all out. It feels like we can't get our head above water. How can we make all this work, and what should we do?

When this happens, it seems the harder we try, the tougher it gets. We are overwhelmed, frustrated, and often angry and exhausted. Our mind is working overtime, searching for solutions to make things work. Our heart hurts; our mind races. We really want to feel good again.

This message came into me during the 1990s. My twenty-three-year marriage ended. It was an amicable ending although still there was great sadness. I had been in a lot of physical pain for several years before this. There were lots of doctor visits and alternative health explorations which started in the 1980s. The unremitting nerve pain resulted in a ruptured cyst, several surgeries, and complete exhaustion. I had always been healthy with good nutrition, exercise, and a loving spiritual practice. So, this was really new to me.

During this time due to my health challenge, I left my position as executive vice president of a wonderful real estate company. The owner, his wife, and their son were and are family to me. It was not an easy decision. However, my health and spirit demanded I explore a new path to restore my health on all levels. It was tough, and I knew it was right.

This was also the time my father's Alzheimer's disease was progressing. My mother was his high school sweetheart, and Mom and I were his caregivers. My heart was hurting for my father's mental turmoil and also for my mother's greatest sadness of her life. Then there was my own hurting heart, as the daughter. My father was a huge inspirational anchor in my life. No matter what I was doing, or what great idea I had next, my dad always told me I would be good at it and just to do my best.

Of course, I was completely out of my Inner River of Peace. It seemed the rapids were rough, and they just kept coming from all directions. I couldn't see which way was forward. There were lots of prayers and good intentions on my part every day. I kept trying hard to make things be better. Being resilient and managing this very stressful season of my life did not seem possible. This only made things tougher and more complicated.

In the throes of all this, in came the wave of peace. As it's always been throughout my life, a wave of peace preceded The Message:

What are you fretting about? Don't you remember?
All YOU agreed to do is:
Show Up and Hold the Vision.
We can do all the rest through you.

Along with The Messenger's Message comes a stillness, a sense of grace.

The struggle and tension started to melt into this peace and stillness. The exhaustion started to vaporize. I was finally moving from my desert of isolation back to my Inner River of Peace. There is always a calm reassurance and sometimes a strange sense of wonder. On a spiritual level, it reminds me of how a cool glass of water feels when I'm really hot and thirsty on a physical level. It feels like the nectar of God.

The peace and stillness of The Message bring a sense that everything is okay. Everything will be okay. And no matter what happens, it will still be okay. Nature shows us there are calm waters after the rapids. There is spring after winter. We can't avoid the rapids of life. However, we can create tools of resilience and wisdom for managing the stress. Then we are creatively strengthening our spirit and body. There is some feeling of being back in some sort of self-control. Feeling completely out of control is a big part of these very tough experiences in our life.

I still remember the sense of peace that permeated every fiber of my being when The Message came through me. The tightness dissolved with the assurance I was not alone. I did not have to figure this out for myself. What a welcomed realization and sense of relief. These comforting thoughts and feelings simultaneously sent corresponding biochemical brain signals to receptor sites on cells throughout my body. The physiological shift was a palpable sense of relief. The body was reminded to ease up. Everything is going to be okay, somehow.

This Message took me back to my Inner River of Peace. Oh, how I wanted to hold on to this place forever. It was a big breath of fresh air. My sense of well-being was getting restored.

My job was twofold: to keep showing up and to keep holding the vision for the guidance, wisdom, and peace for how I could function better. I wanted to be strong to help my father and mother. The Message reminded me that I was the vessel, and the vessel was needed as a physical conduit. Without the vessel, there was nothing there to receive the guidance and take the action. We are the vessel, the vehicle, and the instrument that is needed in this world of physical matter and form. We can become part of the peace of which we all yearn. Our mental and emotional energy is where it all originates. The peace and balance we yearn for starts with our thoughts and feelings. This is reflected in our words and actions. We must trust in the gentle power of the flow (poem in Review 7-9).

There was a calm quietness in knowing, if I showed up and held the vision, I would be shown the way forward. It would come to me when I needed it. I knew I must trust this, if I wanted to survive and keep one foot anchored in my Inner River of Peace, while the other foot handled the activity in the physical world of happenings. Some part of us knows this is possible. Thus, hope can prevail in the most seemingly impossible situations.

Interpretation

What does "Showing Up" mean to you?

Showing up is something we do for our heart and our mind. It can be physical or nonphysical. If it refers to an event, then, of course, we must physically show up while holding the vision of the desired intention. If it's a desire for a specific outcome, like guidance or clarity on a topic, then we show up by holding the vision in our thoughts and prayers. Quiet time, prayer, and meditation are meaningful examples of showing up in the nonphysical way. Tai chi, qigong, and yoga are among many meaningful contemplative practices in the physical way.

Showing up is claimed to be as much as 90% of a result. You have already done this. You are here right now reading The Message with me and others. Even when we least feel like it, we know if we can just get our self to show up, something can happen. The odds are in our favor.

So, just keep showing up with The Message for seven days or your desired length of time. Relate it to your situation and vision. You are making this Message your own as you bring it into your life as much as possible. Incorporate it into things you are already doing. Each time you repeat The Message in a situation, slow down and be still. Simply be aware of what showing up means for you.

Having The Message in your day serves to restore a healthy sense of well-being. There is comfort here. After all, when you show up in *your* Inner River of Peace, the river will take you where you are to go. That power greater than us guides our way home to this river.

Have you noticed? Sometimes when we show up for one reason, we find out that a completely different reason was what it was really all about. We would not have found this other great thing if we had not shown up for the first thing. Things are not always as they seem.

Example: I thought I was showing up on an airplane with my mother for the sole reason of flying to my brother and sister-in-law's home to bury our father's ashes. However, next to my mother was seated a man who was amazingly sweet with my mother. They spoke to each other during most of the flight. I married him one year later. Now who created that situation?

Do you remember Dr. Seuss's children's book *Oh, the Places You'll Go!?* This is a good time to read it again. It's one of my favorite re-reads throughout life. It's like The Messages. The wisdom keeps ringing true throughout our lives. We must keep showing up and carrying on, through the thick, scary, dark forests of our life's journey. The sun shines, the sky opens up, and the river clears eventually. After all, the dark of winter is followed by the light of spring.

What does "Hold the Vision" mean to you?

"Vision: an act or power of the imagination." *Webster's New World Dictionary.*

Imagination is more important than knowledge.
Albert Einstein

Show Up and Hold the Vision

There are no limits on our imagination, dreams, and visions. There are many kinds of visions: big ones and little ones. They can be specific, general, or ongoing prayer-visions. Having a vision means holding our focus with our thinking heart and feeling mind on an ideal, a desire, something we really want to bring into being.

Specific visions are for a person, place, or thing.

Example: Your vision for the good outcome of a meeting, phone call, event, doctor's appointment, your child's day at school, or your current dream-project.

General visions are for clarity, guidance, and more trust for wherever we are. Often, we cannot see the beautiful forest through the huge trees.

Example: Clarity for the right place to work or live, the right time to do something, the right way to handle a caregiving situation that seems impossible. This helps when we are in overwhelm and need some guidance and love to soothe our hurting heart.

Ongoing prayer-visions are *those for the evolving Path of Our Personal Legend.* (Paulo Coelho). These visions are great support for accomplishing an ongoing sense of purpose or the fruition of a dream.

Example: Your continued good health getting better and better on all levels every day, your desire to practice the Presence of God during your day, your wish to be a more peaceful and compassionate person, your search for your purpose, or your long-term dreams and goals.

Holding the vision for writing this book is an example of my ongoing prayer-vision that finally came into form. I held the vision in my heart and mind for many decades and held onto the dream-goal. It also held onto me and would not let me go. The process called for patience and waiting for divine timing, divine order, and divine grace to come along.

Stop and look right now. Don't get overwhelmed with ideas. Ease up on yourself. Listen to one vision that's true for you right now. Choose something that is really in your heart. Explore this specific vision for seven days or something better. Ask for the guidance. As you do this, you build your heart-mind muscle. Then showing up and holding your vision becomes a natural creative process in your life for creating your current vision. With focus and use over time, this mode of operandi becomes programmed into your autonomic nervous system. We are now becoming more resilient when struggle and stress raise their persistent heads. The Messenger comes to the rescue, for our asking, thinking, doing, and being.

Holding the vision means you are holding the power for goodness and peace to prevail. It does not mean we just show up and simply sit there. Take it on with the excited hopeful eyes of a child expecting a present with a sense of wonder. Metaphorically release your clenched fists and keep your hands open to receive. Something might come in much better than you thought you wanted. Don't miss the beautiful boat, while you are wishing for a life raft.

This is an active Message, not a passive one. We must plant the seed, water it, and love it with all our heart and spirit. The mind will follow. Then, there is the wait and see part. The timing of The Message's wisdom is not usually in our desired timeframe. Patience in holding the vision and waiting for the results is seldom a top human attribute.

Divine timing is in a world of its own. If we wait for it, we don't have to go back and fix the situation later. This calls for trust and lots of faith. Our ability to trust with faith builds over time and strengthens the heart-mind muscle. It's waiting for us to exercise it, and it loves to be strong and courageous, as it gives us a new way to think and feel. This liberation is exhilarating.

Our reward for showing up and holding the vision is a more peaceful way to live. We get better at this all the time with practice. Commit to the focus of holding the vision for all the guidance and love available for you. Decide not to get discouraged, and if you do, bring your heart and mind back to your vision. You can learn to trust and love this new way of being and doing. Anchor deep in *your* Inner River of Peace. Honor the wisdom of divine timing.

Increase your awareness and find your best times and ways to repeat The Message during your daily happenings, such as when you are:

- Getting up in the morning
- Brushing your teeth
- Taking yourself or your dog for a walk
- Pausing to look at whatever nature is available
- Doing chores and errands
- Resolving a problem
- Going to appointments, classes, or events
- Enjoying coffee or teatime
- Taking a bath
- Turning out the light at night
- Laying your head on the pillow

Show Up and Hold the Vision

What we do daily, keeps creating who we are now and who we are becoming in the future. Wherever you are in your life and whatever you are doing, hold the vision of seeing good results. Often there are quite pleasant surprises. Remember to reflect and be full of thanks. The more we do this, the more it happens. Our Inner River of Peace is brimming with amazing adventures.

Know that *your* Inner River of Peace is always there. You are now in the process of fine-tuning your ability to stay connected to it. Life is a challenging adventure. Look at the challenges and courageous things you have done before. Let them strengthen your heart-mind muscle and feel the inspiration. Trust yourself like never before. This starts with showing up and holding the vision for the wisdom and love The Messenger has for you.

Our body is a temple for our heart and soul. It is also a chemistry tube of physical elements and nonphysical thoughts, memories, and emotions. It sizzles and pops constantly with everything we do and think, while it strives to maintain homeostasis. This is the body's way of keeping the Inner River of Peace flowing.

We don't always know what to expect or what the answer is. Despite the fear and anxiety of the unknown, we can learn to trust The Messenger to lead us back to our Inner River of Peace. If you are not willing to *Show Up and Hold the Vision*, you will miss out on some very rich life experiences. Courage is part of this Message.

Message One

Heroism is the dazzling and glorious concentration of courage.
Henri-Frederic Amiel

May we be dazzling and glorious with our courage every day. Think of a time when you did this in your life. Be empowered by that courageous action. Pull up that empowered feeling and focus on it like a magnifying glass. Concentration is magnification, and form will follow.

My dazzling courageous memory: My brother, Peter, was a professional river runner, serving as a river guide in raft trips through the Grand Canyon and down the Green and Colorado Rivers. My sister, Sally, and I took one of his amazing seven-day trips with our husbands and two other couples. There were two small rafts. Each raft had two couples and one guide. Peter and his fellow guide, Neal, were our leaders. I was excited and a bit anxious. We were going to be navigating Cataract Canyon, known as one of the most dangerous navigable rapids in the United States.

It was thrilling to travel for seven days on small rafts through the Canyonlands. We camped on the riverbanks in sleeping bags under the stars, and cooked meals over the open fire. Each night we gathered wood and built the fire inside a fire pan we laid on the ground for environmental reasons. The cherry pie in a Dutch-oven was the best pie we ever had! The morning coffee was the best coffee we ever had, too. Each campsite looked untouched when we

Show Up and Hold the Vision

left each morning to ride the river to the next evening's site. Every campsite was a meaningful experience in this cathedral of nature.

I remember the anticipation and the fear I felt in my gut when we came to the Cataract Canyon rapids on one of the last days. The raging rapids were heard but could not be seen. They dropped below the river's horizon and sounded like a roaring freight train. To add to the excitement, it was raining with some thunder and lightning. For more excitement, I had horrible cramps in my stomach. Between the storm and the ice-cold river, we were all soaking wet and frozen to the bone.

Just before entering the rapids, Peter and Neal pulled the rafts over to the side of the river and the eight of us got out. Sitting on the riverbank, we watched Peter and Neal up on a rock reading the river. Into the rafts we went. First slowly and quietly, we drifted with guidance towards the horizon as our river guides stood up for a few moments intensely focused on the horizon's entry point. In a split second, they sat down and paddled ferociously towards the horizon of thunderous sounds. They were dazzlingly focused on the spot on the horizon for the desired entry point of the rapids. Hitting that desired spot with the raft was crucial to surviving the rapids. The goal was to avoid Devil's Hole.

My teeth were chattering with fright and cold, and it felt like my stomach was up against my spine. The call for courage came in as we barreled down the river towards the rapids. Saddling up was the only choice, so I dug deep and got a grip as I turned my head and focused my eyes on the horizon. There was no turning back now. Forward we went, entering the rapids at just the right point on the horizon line and dropping off into a roaring river.

It was a river-ride adventure of a lifetime. Being tossed in rapids is a surefire way to experience the power of water. Waves were coming over our heads from all directions as Peter skillfully guided the raft through Cataract Canyon. Peter was yelling, "Bail, bail," or more like "Bail, damn it, bail," as we hung onto the ropes with one hand, while the other hand attempted to hang onto the bucket and bail.

At last, the river cleared in the silent stillness of calm waters. There were exuberant shouts of Yee Ha and jumps for joy. We survived. I was thrilled, full of adrenalin, and wanted to do it again.

Look at the exhilarating experience and amazing memory I would have missed if I had not shown up and held the vision for this adventure dream trip of a lifetime. And now the story is here for you.

You don't have to take a river trip to be thrilled or chilled to the bone. There is always something that requires mustering up our glorious courage that dazzles the heartstrings.

Show Up and Hold the Vision

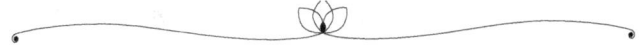

Ideas and Actions

See how much you can enjoy living with The Message for a week or something better. Our heart's desire is to live our lives as much as possible in our Inner River of Peace. This increases our resilience in handling stress. What could be a better use of our time and energy while we are here?

Show Up and Hold the Vision

Place The Message somewhere that keeps it in your line of sight. Add it to your journal, phone, iPad, or keep it on an index card. Have it in a reminder that pops up at certain times of the day. Record the date and your current situation along with any wisdom that comes through for you. There might be several different times it comes forth to assist you in different circumstances. As a universal truth for all of us, The Message applies personally to your unique time and place in life.

While making The Message part of a *holy habit*, little by little you begin to make it yours. Give it time to speak to your thinking heart and feeling mind that are being expanded. Now you are developing your heart-mind muscle. Together, they create a powerful sacred synergy. Our spirit dances with delight when these two parts of us work together. They become a highly effective performance team beyond our wildest imagination.

Stop, Look, and Listen (SLL) as you *Show Up and Hold the Vision.*

Slow, Still, and Simple (SSS) as you wait for the light bulb of wisdom to shine through.

Pause, repeat this often. Notice and observe what's happening. Be open to how The Message speaks to your situation. It's a gift that keeps giving throughout your life at the most interesting and fascinating times.

Read through the chapter, *The Power of the 5 Senses Plus 2,* and select one idea to combine with The Message. Integrating one of the senses when reviewing The Message, takes it beyond the intellect and deeper into your being on a cellular and energetic level.

Example: Be still and breathe for a few minutes when sipping your wonderful cup of coffee or tea. Smell the aroma with thoughts of The Message.

Essential oil example: Simply take 3-5 deep breaths from a bottle of pure lavender, only if you love lavender *(Lavandula augustifolia)*. This is a fast track to your brain and a portal to *your* Inner River of Peace. Orange *(Citrus sinensis)* is another option.

Show Up and Hold the Vision

Choose an aroma that soothes your scattered mind
and speaks to your heart.

You might like to do this with another person for added inspiration. It's interesting to hear their vision and resulting wisdom. Perceptions are widened and set free from their mental box.

Bringing our scattered parts back together is one of the main missions of our Inner River of Peace. From here we are able to connect to the River of Peace in others. With this comes the consciousness that we all meet as one in the Big River of Peace. We know rivers empty into oceans. In the great ocean of existence, we find a reverence for life in all things great and small. We realize we are not alone.

On some level, perhaps we all agreed to show up here and play our part on the stage of life. We want to be part of the peace in the world. What we have in us is what we give to others. We can't give away what we don't have. The more we build our true selves up, the stronger connection we have with our Inner River of Peace.

Message One

Contemplative Moments

Three Steps of Vision-Making

Engage your heart-mind muscle while sensing with your vision.

1. Set the desire and prayer for your vision.
2. Focus on it daily while showing up with your heart-mind muscle for a week. Choose one sensory idea. See chapter, *The Power of the 5 Senses Plus 2*.
3. Release your tight grip on what you think needs to happen. Let the power much greater than all of us show you what it has, while doing steps 1 and 2. Be curious.

Three-Step Prayer

Repeat any time to enhance The Message.

1. May I increase my awareness to receive the **Guidance**.
2. May I have the **Courage** to follow the wisdom when I get the Guidance.
3. May I do this with the kind of **Faith** that moves mountains.

Simple Focused-Breathing Technique

Do anywhere, like standing in the grocery line.

1. **Breathe in** through your nose, while saying/thinking, **I am Showing Up.**

   Pause and be still.

Your Inner River of Peace

2. **Breathe out** through your mouth, while saying, **and I am Holding the Vision for** _____ (insert your vision).

   Pause and be still again.
3. Repeat at least three times. Give thanks ahead of time, every breath of the way.

Once in a While Remember To:

Stop, Look, and Listen (SLL)
Ask yourself what's really going on?

Slow, Still, and Simple (SSS)
How can you bring more ease into your life?

The most beautiful thing we can experience is the mysterious.
It is the source of all true art and science.
Albert Einstein

Be aware of the mysterious beauty The Messenger reveals to you through Message One. *The Power of the 5 Senses Plus 2,* holds more mysterious and beautiful ideas to add to The Message.

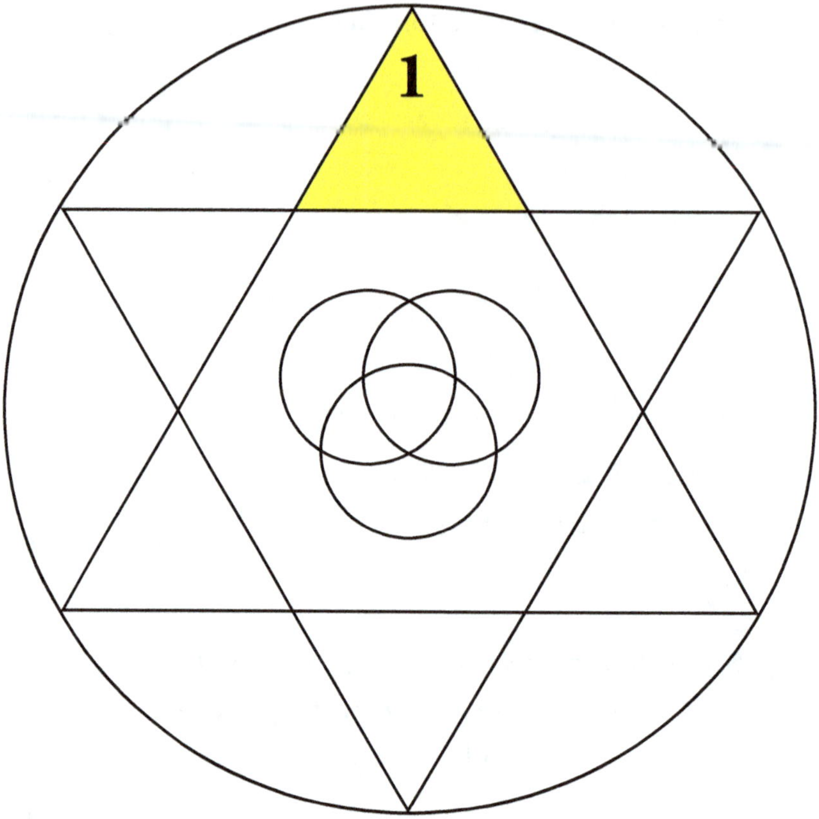

Message One

Message One:

*What are you fretting about? Don't you remember?
All YOU agreed to do is:
Show Up and Hold the Vision.
We can do all the rest through you.*

Your Inner River of Peace

Message Two
Look at the Sky

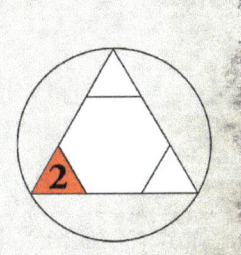

The Message

*Whenever you Think you are limited,
Look at the sky.*

In other words, thinking you are limited is only in your thinking mind. Take the lid off your head-box and know that all things are possible on some level somewhere. Look up at the unlimited space of the sky and the stars. Dreams and miracles are waiting and available for you. Think with your heart and move your heart-mind muscle into the field of unlimited possibilities. Who are we to say something is possible or not?

Be still for one breath right now. Think back on one awesome view of the sky that you loved. If you can go look at the sky right now, wherever you are, just observe it. Repeat The Message. There are no limitations out there, day or night, sunshine or darkness.

The sky displays the stars of the universe to us. They shine, they move, they sparkle, they change. So it is, and so do we.

My Personal Story

In the early 1990s, we ended up living in a small little home in Naples, Florida, that we had owned as a rental property. We had just lost the ownership of our tennis club and our home. Thus, we needed a place to live. When the tenants lease was up, we knew we had to move in. There is a time for all seasons, and this too shall pass.

This rental home turned into a sweet little rescue-sanctuary. Our carpenter friend did all the repairs and remodel in return for tennis lessons. This was nothing short of a miracle. He added an outdoor private deck with a garden and outdoor shower. Since the kitchen was all torn up by tenants, it became the dining area. The old porch turned into the new kitchen with windows looking onto this secret garden. The one mile walk to the beach was a saving grace for me. Being around water is one of the best healing elements. Our bodies are mainly water; no wonder we can feel happy simply by looking at it.

I had just joined the John R. Wood Properties in Naples, launching into my next career. The owner, his wife, and son were like family to me, and I have always loved real estate. Looking at homes, land, and buildings, with eyes of how to improve them, was one of my naturally creative day-dreaming pastimes. Our real estate investments were the reason we had this house that transformed into a sweet little rescue-sanctuary home in which to live, recover, lick our wounds, and eventually thrive again.

So, I had now gone from being a tennis professional-club owner to a real estate salesperson. Needless to say, the anxiety and identity confusion was painfully real. I immediately started taking courses to master this field of work. One of the best was the Dale Carnegie course on public speaking, business, and relationships. Yes, you can say I was completely pushing the boundaries of my comfort zone. One of these evening classes before making my speech, I was sure I was either going to faint or throw-up.

Joining a gym with physical workouts everyday was an important part of this transition. It flushed the stress out of my body and helped to build my sense of self-worth and self-confidence. My body went from an athletic career to one that could have been quite sedentary. These workouts were part of my restoration plan. They helped me spiritually and emotionally make the transition and heal from big losses. My spiritual practice and the power of prayer were foundational anchors for everything.

After a while, I realized my routine at the gym had become a *holy habit*. My spirit was strengthening, and my physical body was getting restored too. It was so important to my entire sense of well-being that it became a daily fix. Pumping oxygen through my body and shifting my brain chemistry fed each cell in my body to rejuvenate in a healthy and positive way. My cellular activity was getting new messages of strength and regeneration.

So, yes, you can imagine the mental challenge my mind was throwing at me with the wild monkeys of negative thinking trying to prevail. I have always loved getting up high and looking around. It can lift my spirits and bring in moments of serenity. The little sanctuary-home had a slightly pitched roof which served as a healthy slant board. I called Home Depot and asked if they had a ladder and if they would deliver it. The ladder came and up against the house it went. I had my way to the roof and my pathway to the sky.

At the end of the day in my favorite evening times, I would climb my ladder of trust to the rooftop of possibilities. Laying there upside down (just a little pitch) looking at the sky was a real treat in several ways. This gave my body a slant board for physical gravity-relief, and it was calming to the nonphysical emotions. One particular evening, I was watching the treetops, the energy light rings glowing around them, and the beautiful blue endless sky beyond them. The clouds were materializing, changing forms, and vaporizing as they passed. I was thinking how life is like this, too. I thought I had lost my connection to The Messages. By the grace of God, in came the calm wave of peace ushering in The Message.

Whenever you Think you are limited,
Look at the sky.

The moment-in-time stillness followed. It felt like a glimpse of grace. I felt the comfort from this Message connecting me to my deep Inner River of Peace that I believed was always somewhere within me. I sensed everything was really okay right now and would continue to be okay, no matter what happened.

The gratitude for this kind of experience and for this Message of universal truth (for all of us) brings the kind of love that takes us to our knees. There is a stillness and simplicity that most of life and the nonsense of the world does not provide or encourage. Our role is to let the clouds of thoughts and emotions float by and focus on the blue sky that eventually prevails. There is a time for all seasons. Nature promises us that seasons do change. Sometimes, it just doesn't follow our narrow idea of time.

Message Two

You are the sky. The clouds are what happens,
what comes and goes.
Eckhart Tolle

Resistance drains our energy and it creates more struggle and pain. Let's focus on being like the sky. It adapts to everything. Its colors are brilliant. Its reservoir is endless.

By the way, I went on to be one of the top salespersons after three years of slowly doing it my way. I read all the success books and tapes on how to be successful in real estate. Yet, I knew that I had to be who I was and do it my way to feel good about myself and truly help people. It took me three years to get to the top. I was then invited to be on the Board of Directors, and after eight years of top sales, I became the Executive Vice President of John R. Wood Properties. It is still a privately/family owned company and one of the most prestigious in the world. I traveled to Hawaii for a national convention, and to Switzerland for the Estates Club International Meeting. Some events in our lives do go way beyond our wildest dreams.

Ten years earlier, I would never have believed this was in my future. I had clients that I loved like family. Taking care of them and having them trust me was a perfect purpose for me. My job was to educate them, help them think, and show them their options.

Look at the Sky

I continue to call in this universal Message of Love throughout my life.

Whenever you Think you are limited,
Look at the sky.

Think and realize all the times in your life, or even in one day, that this Message can ring true for you. It can mentally release some struggle, fear, and confusion. The body will follow the mind's lead. The grip of our frustrations loosens, and we function with more clarity. Search for the unique wisdom for your situation.

The Messenger is always there for us. Our awareness and willingness to be open to receive The Message is paramount. This connection builds faith and trust. We are innately connected to The Messenger. This is a good time to practice building our heart-mind muscle by thinking with our hearts and feeling with our minds. We get better and better at trusting this the more we *Show Up and Hold the Vision* for our ability to do so. Being on our knees once in a while and being full of thanksgiving, aligns us with the beauty in our true self in many ways.

Message Two

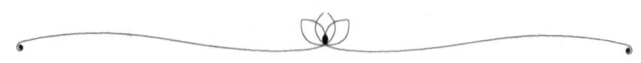

Interpretation

What does "Whenever you Think you are limited" mean to you?

We can feel limited in many ways. It may be a physical limitation from birth or from an event in our life. It can be mental and emotional from our chemical make-up, or from past tough experiences, current challenges, or future fears. This is all part of the human dilemma. Part of our purpose in life is to really understand who we are as our unique magnificent self. There is no one else on the planet like us. May we embrace who we are, and see how well we can live each day, and be resilient as we go through life. Believe and realize it is possible to move on and thrive. The seemingly death of winter always turns into the blossoms of spring. Do you believe you can trust this for sure in life challenges? We are part of the rhythms and cycles of nature. What a blessing. Let us remember this.

First, we want to realize the reason that makes us *Think* we are limited. If it's physical, look to others with similar situations that have persevered. Also observe how others who, so far in their life, have not been able to persevere. They all serve as inspiration and reminders to encourage us to decide how we want to think and feel with new dreams and desires. With decisions come new thoughts, new feelings, and new words. Also, new thoughts and new feelings create new decisions and new actions. These profound experiences shift our current and future path.

Our thoughts create who we are and who we will become on many levels. They reveal the possibilities, even when we think there is no way out. Being in the overwhelming seemingly impossible throes of caregiving is an example of this. I know, I have been there, too.

One time I ended up in the hospital with chest pains. This was a big wake-up call for giving myself some nurturing. If I didn't take care of myself, who would help my dad with Alzheimer's and Mom helping Dad? If I go down, then I would need someone to care for me. A conundrum to say the least.

When I got out of the hospital, I went away for a week to a Prayer House in the respite of the Appalachian Mountains. Mom had mentioned this place to me months before the hospital event. The importance of this cannot be overstated. It reconnected me to my Inner River of Peace. That is what I could be for my mom and dad.

Sometimes the reason we think we are limited is initially not physical. This might include a troubled past, an overload of exhaustion, or depression and anxiety. We humans are amazing. Observe those who anchored deep and met their personal challenge and thrived. We can overcome hurdles with incredible strength.

Message Two

Our Inner River of Peace is always deep inside of us somewhere. Use The Message to carry you back home to this river. The unique wisdom for you is wrapped in the power of a gentle comforter of love and trust.

Perhaps we've had a feeling of failure of one kind or another. Even though failure can be a steppingstone to success, it doesn't feel that way when we're in the middle of the cacophony. The truth is we were successful in having the courage to try something we wanted to do. We won't have to regret we didn't try it as age eighty in a rocking chair. However, it still can feel devastating and be accompanied by total exhaustion.

The body may also be challenged with a compromised immune system, nervous system, and all the rest of our amazing systems. They are all interconnected, so we can't keep it isolated to one system. Stress knows no limits in affecting our whole self. This presents quite the challenge. Now, we don't have the energy to boost ourselves up. So, we saddle up and anchor deep, and call in our Inner River of Peace. Getting any help needed keeps us going, one drop and one step at a time.

> *The marvelous richness of human experience would lose*
> *something of rewarding joy*
> *if there were no limitations to overcome.*
> Helen Keller

Look at the Sky

Wherever the mind goes, the body follows. Wherever our heart goes, our minds will follow. Our minds are brilliant and have a connection to the endless field of unlimited possibilities. Our mind can be our best or not-best friend. We can also see it as a magical kingdom of healing and creation. Let's embrace our heart and mind for the fertile field they create together. The thought-seeds we plant start here. We have a lifetime to plant seeds and nurture this potential field of abundance. It is an integral part of our Inner River of Peace. Honoring who we are is part of our life's purpose. This means we must be honest with ourselves.

Part of the human dilemma is to continue to strengthen our ability to shift the scarcity mentality to our desired abundance mentality. This is part of the royal mission these Messages reveal to us. Prosperity comes in many shapes and forms.

Perhaps we have a life purpose and dream that keeps yearning to materialize. Maybe we think we're limited with our life situation, and this purpose is just not going to get fulfilled. Read and talk to people who have done this. Surround yourself as much as possible with people, places, and things that support you and bring up the realm of inspiration. Grab your Message and keep it close. Plant this seed of guidance and wisdom in your heart and mind. When they work together, the love affair creates abundant life.

Our role is to keep our focus on the possibility of unlimited potential. With our mind out of its comfortable box, we can trust the power beyond and within us. Why would we want to think otherwise when we can choose these thoughts? Why would we want to keep dragging ourselves around in the desert of struggle, anger, and frustration, when we can make the pilgrimage back to the oasis of lush foliage, sweet dates, and wells of pure spring water? Our Inner River of Peace is an oasis.

As we learn and practice *thinking* with our heart and *feeling* with our mind, we realize they can create a highly effective performance team. Instead of struggling with each other, they actually assist one another in a brilliant way in the challenging adventures of our life.

I decided to do this when my frustration and struggle between my mind and soul resulted in a few nightmares in my dreamtime. The pain led me to the survival mode of deeper prayers and imagination. I envisioned my mind and heart recognizing each other for the brilliant elements they are, and how they could release the turmoil. I imagined my heart and mind in a virtual marriage, having a great love affair of unencumbered joy. Our spirit dances with delight anytime the heart and mind finally get together. Even for a fleeting moment in time, it's a good practice. Each time we do this, we get better for future opportunities to practice again.

Look at the Sky

Take a moment and imagine how your life would look if your heart and mind embraced and honored each other, empowered by your soul and spirit. The mental thoughts would be checked and balanced by the heart's wisdom. The feeling heart would be checked and balanced by the mind's love. The resulted synergy of each of their strengths would be harmony in thought, feeling, words, and actions. Now this is really something we can sink our teeth into and continue to master. As long as we are here, the mastery isn't totally completed. However, life provides us with plenty of experiences to practice building this relationship and keep reaping the rewards.

Stop, Look, and Listen (SLL).

What are the limiting thoughts?

Slow, Still, and Simple (SSS).

How can you think and feel differently with your heart and mind working together?

Make a secret promise to yourself that makes you feel good and gives you hope. Keep taking one breath and one sacred step at a time. Eventually, Spring arrives in its own time.

What does "Look at the sky" bring up for you?

The sky is available to all of us, even when we can't see it. The sky is always there with its ever-flowing freedom without boundaries. All we have to do is look at it. We can see the sky; we can only imagine the sky's world of possibilities.

Message Two

As we all wander around down here on planet earth, humans have always looked to the sky with a childlike sense of wonder. The stars and the moon have been respites for our wearied souls. Astrology has guided the path of humans from the beginning of existence. Gazing at the sky and the universe provides gateways into our imagination and dreams. They serve as an unbounded source of inspiration.

The freedom of flight comes to my mind. Look at the people who against all odds, envisioned and invented hot air balloons, airplanes, and spaceships. It didn't always happen in their lifetime, but it happened. Leonardo da Vinci created the drawings for many of these in the 1400s. Inventions start with a dream and a belief. The creators of these inventions knew they were not limited in their thoughts and actions of creation. It took time and relentless commitment to the vision and the dream. The sky was always there to remind them. All they had to do was *Look at the Sky* and imagine.

Whenever I fly in airplanes, I love to have a window seat, so I can just gaze out and into the beyond. Usually it is a great source of tranquility. Some of my best ideas and insights come in from this form of gazing. It's awesome and mysterious looking into the sky from afar. This sense of freedom and liberation is a good space to

Look at the Sky

be in whenever we get the opportunity. Look for places like this for you—or just *Look at the Sky*.

I love to go out in the early morning and later in the night with our dog. As she does her business and checks around for smells, I gaze at the sky. It's never the same: light, dark, moon, stars, clear, or cloudy. Whether the time is early or late, daytime or nighttime, the sky is a masterpiece of colors, smells, sights, and sounds. Our life is a masterpiece too when we consciously decide with our heart-mind muscle to believe it. As Wayne Dyer said, "We'll see it when we believe it."

Stop and look out at the vastness of nature. It speaks to us if we listen. The sky is a metaphor for vast fields of infinity. On the earth we have oceans, deserts, and the wide-open spaces of fields and flat ranges that reach to the horizon. I have a memory of driving across Kansas, as well as the deserts of the southwest. There are memories of the majestic beauty of the mountain-top ranges going on as far as the eye can see.

There are several times in my life when I found myself in the clouds. Two of them were above the cloud line at the top of the Andes in Ecuador and in Peru. When the clouds came in, they completely engulfed me. There were only a few feet of visibility. When they cleared, the view of endless mountaintops went on as far as I could see.

Message Two

Clouds and storms come and go, like challenges in our lives. There is a natural order in the seasons of the days and years of our lives. Every time the clouds of life arrive, we are called to anchor deep and trust. When the clouds of life pass, the sky is still there. And so it is, with the Inner River of Peace.

Look at people who have refused to go down with the limited mentality state that so often comes with certain life events. Look at the people who refused to let go of their dreams, visions, and purpose. Inspiration comes just thinking about these people, reminding us to keep looking up.

Hold on to your vision, small or large. It could be the desire to simply get through the day in front of you with love and compassion. A deepening trust in divine timing is part of showing up and holding the vision. Knowing you are not limited and looking at the sky brings hope. This lifts our spirit out of the heavy dross of the moment.

The time it takes to get a nonphysical vision or dream into the physical form of matter is part of the great unknown. It's always easy to get ideas of success and things we want to create and do. Bringing them into form is a whole other state of existence. It might come in on the next phone call, or it might take decades. *Your* Inner River of Peace will help you hold onto hope and build more faith. Smooth flowing waters sustain us. Thus, The Message guides you to

Look at the Sky

your Inner River of Peace through this adventure called life, as an integral and powerfully important part of your dreams and visions. Your dream may simply be to have more peace in your life. What would that take?

Remember to *Show Up and Hold the Vision* of your dreams and purpose (little or big), and *Whenever you Think you are limited, Look at the Sky*. There are no limits on our imagination. The ability within each of us to keep going is an inspiring power to explore. This power is greater than anything we can imagine.

Imagination and inspiration are words that make us feel good just thinking about them. Explore their possibilities with The Messages.

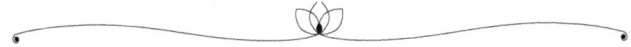

Ideas and Actions

Feel some peace just knowing you have The Message with you. Find the best way for you to keep this message in your heart and mind. Add the words to your computer, device, phone or any place you will look at often. Your car, the bathroom mirror, and your wallet are options. Put it in a pocket close to your heart. Be creative.

Message Two

> *Whenever you Think you are limited,*
> *Look at the sky.*

This Message can serve you well throughout life. Consider keeping a record of the situation you are in and any wisdom that is revealed.

Whether you use this message for a week or another way, set the intention to get all the goodness and wisdom it has for you at this time and situation in your life. The longer length of time you use it, the more you will see how it assists you on deeper levels throughout life. It can become part of your autonomic nervous system response. Then you receive the wisdom, not only on the intellectual plane, but also on the cellular level. Your heart-mind muscle is empowered again.

If you like to write, draw, or paint, set up a journal for these Messages of Love. Make your own coloring book with calligraphy lettering. For those of us who love to write, journals are personal and meaningful. Write The Message and your situation. Then record the insights and wisdom that come through for you. If you don't know if you are a writer, be curious and try it. Just find your way that works with The Message. You can find out what this is by asking for it to show itself to you.

> *Whenever you Think you are limited,*
> *Look at the sky.*

Look at the Sky

These *Ten Messages of Love* hold precious golden nuggets for each of us. They are secret hidden treasures that come through at just the right moment. It's important now and then to go against the fast-paced daily den of the world and be:

Slow, Still, and Simple (SSS) to bring The Message into your life as often as you can.

Read through the chapter, *The Power of the 5 Senses Plus 2.* Select one idea to explore with The Message. Choose one you know you love or try a new one that arouses your curiosity.

Example: Whenever you have a favorite treat anytime throughout the day or night, repeat The Message silently or out loud to yourself. You have invited taste to enhance The Message.

Essential oil example: Lemon (*Citrus limonum*) offers its clean clear aroma from up in the trees to lift your spirits. Only if you love it, put 3-4 drops on a cotton ball. Take 3-5 deep breaths and pause with The Message. Keep the cotton ball in a special place, such as your pocket or dish on your desk. Lime, bergamot or grapefruit are other choices. The only requirement here is that you love

Message Two

the aroma. Fruits are in the treetops, reaching for the sky.

Remember, you are developing your heart-mind muscle. This taps into the powerful realm of the soul and spirit, major generators connecting to the Inner River of Peace. Imagine this serving you with a new way to navigate through your life. You have nothing to lose and lots of wisdom and peace to gain. And then there is love.

Look at the Sky

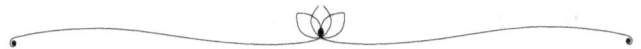

Contemplative Moments

Three Steps of Vision-Making

Engage your heart-mind muscle while sensing with your vision.

1. Set your intention and prayer as you ask The Message for its guidance.
2. Focus on it daily with your heart-mind muscle combined with a sensory action. See the chapter, *The Power of the 5 Senses Plus 2*.
3. Release any tightness in your mind or gut to that precious power greater than us, while you keep doing steps 1 and 2.

Three-Step Prayer

Repeat anytime to enhance The Message.

1. May I increase my awareness to receive the **Guidance.**
2. May I have the **Courage** to follow it when I get it.
3. May I do it with the **Faith** that moves mountains - leaving no room for doubt.

Simple Focused-Breathing Technique

Do anywhere, like standing in the grocery line.

1. **Breathe in** through your nose, while thinking**, Whenever I think I am limited.**

    Pause and be still.

Message Two

2. **Breathe out** through your mouth, while saying, **I Look at the sky.**

    Pause and be still again.
3. Try three of these breaths right now.

    Can you see the sky?

May you be blessed with glimpses of wisdom, insight, and inspiration to increase your Faith as you *Look at the Sky* and know all things are possible. Trusting God is part of my daily intentions. Life is an adventuresome challenge. Being connected with our consciousness to our Inner River of Peace increases our faith.

Faith is the bird that feels the light and sings when the dawn is still and dark.
Rabindranath Tagore

May you be aware of the existence of *your* Inner River of Peace, whether it is day or night, light or dark. It's still there.

Look at the Sky

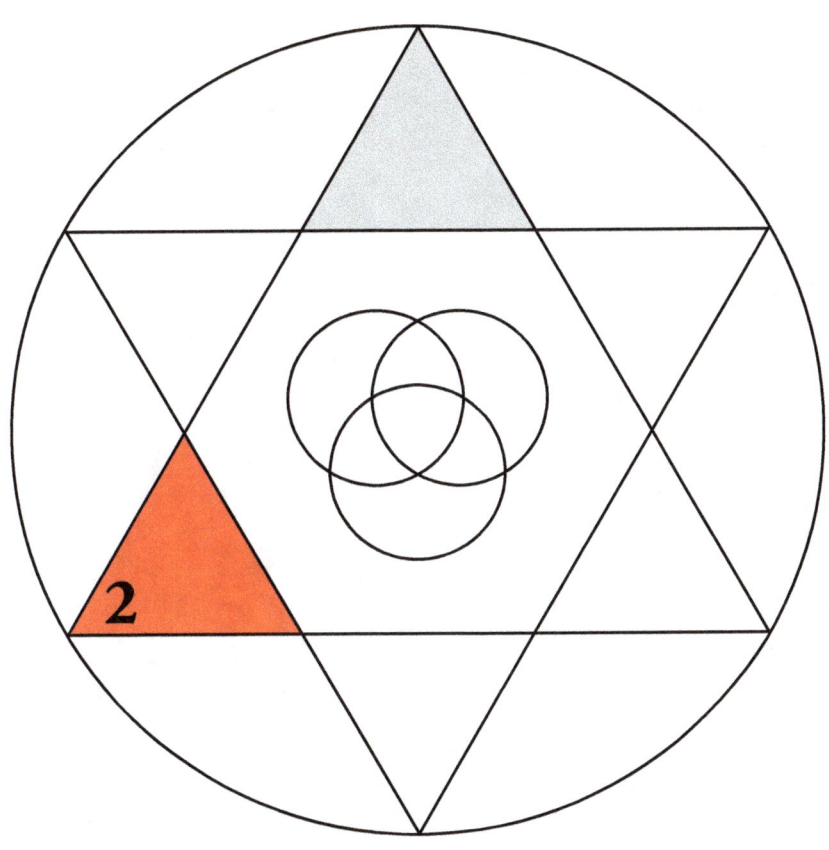

Message Two:

*Whenever you Think you are limited,
Look at the sky.*

MESSAGE THREE
Focus on the Light and Love

The Message

Focus on the Light and the Love and That is what You will magnify.

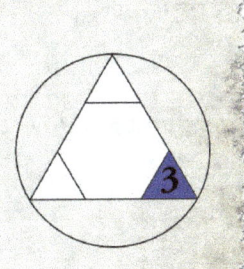

In other words, when the ways of the world shift our minds to scattered thinking, the wild monkeys start having a heyday. It's time to get one foot back into our Inner River of Peace. We can do this by pulling our focus back into the light of our brilliant mind, and the love of our radiant heart.

When we do this, the new thoughts magnify the light that is always there waiting for us to realize it. Our job is to hold the focus. This pointed focus provides the amplification and manifestation of more light and love in many forms. The power out there is much greater than us; however, we are connected to it and part of it. The God Spark is within each us.

Our other big role is to trust ourselves and this power of grace that is ours for the asking, believing, and desiring. Our heart-mind muscle gets stronger. Remember, we are developing our ability to think with our heart and feel with our mind. The harmony created is a treasured gift.

Be still for one breath right now. Your focus is already on some light and love because you are here. Let it in, let it magnify, let it show you the way.

My Personal Story

I love my memory of sitting in solitude in the grotto at the St. Leo Benedictine Abbey in St Leo, Florida. *Webster's New World Dictionary* defines "grotto" as "an artificial cave like structure." They are places of reverence and prayer in quiet nature settings, a refuge from the den of the world.

When I lived in Naples, Florida, periodically I made this 3 ½ hour pilgrimage-drive up to the Abbey, north of Tampa. My usual stays were three nights and three days of prayer and renewal. The reverence of the abbey is palpable. I was brought up in a Methodist church, however, my life experiences have taught me the real basis of true religions and spiritual practices are anchored in the deep river of the love of God.

Sister Lorraine was the innkeeper for the monastery's guesthouse. We become the dearest of friends the very first time we met. Our eyes danced with joy, and we giggled, hugged, and prayed together. She called me her "little sister." Sometimes when I was there, we packed up some food and took a little field trip-excursion for a couple of hours. It was a special time for us.

This particular time, I was there to help her move from her little apartment in the abbey's guesthouse to a room in the monastery prepared for her by the monks. She was getting forgetful and needed supervision with loving eyes watching over her. After getting her moved and settled in with a little welcome party of sweet gifts and treats from the monks, it was time for me to start the trek home. This was the last time I saw her since she passed away shortly after this visit.

As I was pulling out of the entrance, I felt a strong pull to stop at the grotto. It was across the street from the monastery. Every time before, I drove by it and wanted to stop. This time, my car just pulled over. I walked the grounds, and as providence would have it, there was no one else around at all.

Message Three

After wandering through the grotto that was nestled in among a canopy of towering trees, I sat down on a log, gazing around at the beauty of nature. What a sweet time of solitude and rest. All of a sudden, I looked up, and there was an opening high up in the treetops to the sky. The brilliant rays of sunlight came blasting through the opening like a magnifying glass. The Message came in on its wave of peace:

*Focus on the Light and Love
and That is what You will magnify.*

Following the wave of peace, there was a moment in time of stillness embracing me. There was no missing this message. I was grateful for my intuition and the power that turned me and my car into the grotto.

Think what I would have missed, if I hadn't shown up at the monastery that week and held the vision of compassion for those three days. Turning into the grotto for the first time and looking up at the sky, gave me the perfect message of wisdom I needed at that time. I was feeling a bit sad and lonely about Sister Lorraine's situation.

I sat there in reflection, and then headed out for my 3 ½ hour drive home to Naples. The next day was Mother's Day, the day my father passed away two years earlier. Mom and I would go out to lunch and have each other to hug and love.

Little did I know that a few months later, I would be delivering this Message as part of the eulogy I gave for Sister Lorraine's funeral service in the abbey. She was a smiling light in the world who lived this Message. She focused on light and love, with a twinkle in her eye and a joyfulness in her step. This is what she magnified in others.

Brother Gabriel phoned me and said the monks would like me to say a eulogy for her. This was a great leap of faith and a whole new experience for me. Before I could think about it, out of my mouth came: "Yes, I would be honored to give her eulogy." My comfort zone was challenged. I wasn't sure what I was supposed to do. What would I say and how in the world could I stand up there at the pulpit in the monastery?

I saddled up and mustered up my courage to act on this mission I felt called to do. All I knew was that I had to do this for Sister Lorraine. There was no pro-con list to be made. Not doing it was not an option. It's one of those times where you sense that the decision was already made for you. It was an amazing experience of the unknown with some trepidation and finally grace.

After the service, there was more abundance going on. A teenage boy, patiently standing next to me waiting to speak, said he felt I was saying those words just for him. His eyes were full of compassion as he thanked me. I wondered whether I was there just for him. The Mother Superior of Sister Lorraine's Order from France was there. She walked over to me later and said she realized I was the friend Sister Lorraine mentioned to her. She thanked me for saying a eulogy for her. I was humbled and a little glad I didn't know ahead of time the Mother Superior was there.

This is one of those times when all you can do is be grateful. All I did was respond to the call, by saying *Yes*. I showed up, held the vision, and looked up at the sky. That's all we need to do, even if our knees are shaking and our heart is beating a bit faster. Then, we are the vessel for the love beyond our dreams to play through us. Our Inner River of Peace amplifies and prevails. Courage and trust create wonders.

> *You shall see wonders.*
> William Shakespeare

Whatever the call is for your life situation, remember to *Stop, Look, and Listen (SLL)* while you:

> *Focus on the Light and Love*
> *and That is what You will magnify.*

Be curious, explore, and see what happens when you do this for a week or something better. Find the right way for you to use The Message and honor that. The Message will become part of your life to tap into whenever you want or need to focus your heart-mind muscle on it. Here you discover more and become more of your wonderful self. The connection to *your* Inner River of Peace just keeps getting stronger. Simply setting the intention to strengthen this connection is a worthwhile vision for your focus. It serves you well, traveling through life.

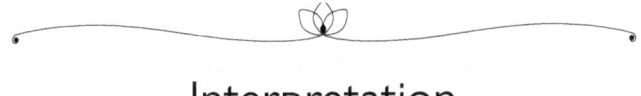

Interpretation

What does "Focus on the Light and Love" mean to you?

"Focus: a central point, the focal point of any system of rays, beams or waves. The point of convergence of the rays is called real focus. The place where a visual image is clearly formed, as in the eye of a camera." *Webster's New World Dictionary*

Just think about the real focus point we can create by putting the rays, beams, and waves of all the parts of who we are on the light and love of our desired outcome. No matter how little or big the vision is, it is of value. If we are not clear on the vision-dream, we will dilute the focus ability.

A scattered or diluted focus tends to create unrest, confusion, and a fried nervous system. However, when we embrace this non-clarity, it becomes part of the process of honing our focus. This calls for perspective and realization. It is a good reason to keep your focus on finding the wisdom this Message has for you.

Focus is a word we hear a lot that is applicable to just about every situation we encounter. Think about where your focus goes most of the day. Is it on the past actions and emotions that don't make you feel good? This prevents us from being in the present. Some of these thoughts and feelings can be regrets, frustration, or anger.

Doubts and fears of the future get in the way of our ability to *Focus on the Light and Love.* This is part of the human dilemma. These can be thoughts and memories of the past we are afraid will happen again. Fear effects our sense of self-worth and self-confidence in moving forward. What are your fears of the future? Some are the fears of success or the fears of failure or just flat-out fear of the unknown. If we lay down our fears and doubts of the future, just think of what we can create. There is a point where enough light and love will melt away the fears and doubts.

Each day we get another chance to refuse to focus on the worries. With a new focus, we can shift our thoughts and feelings to some light and love in today. Visions we love for the future get revived by our gratitude for today. When Pooh Bear asked Christopher Robin what day it was, Christopher said: *"It is today."* Pooh Bear replied: *"Oh, Good! Today is my favorite day!"*

Focus on the Light and Love

Every day we awaken is today. Rain or shine, we choose our mental focus the best we can. I love Pooh Bear's words of wisdom. It's on a post-it on the top of my laptop right now. It lifts my spirit about being in today just by looking at it. We need these reminders because the mind likes to wander off into the past or future or the dross of the world. Let The Message help you pull your focus back into today.

A telescope, microscope, camera lenses or cross hairs in a scope change the way we see things, and they can change our life. Have you noticed the laser focus of an animal? I watch our precious chocolate lab-mix doggie, Muga, when she spots something moving or watches her ball I have just thrown. She sits there waiting for my command to go get it. Her eyes never leave the ball that has landed in the grass. Muga teaches me great stuff.

Muga came into our life from the Humane Society in Pagosa Springs, Colorado, at three months of age. We named her Muga, a Japanese word that means *to be completely absorbed in a peak experience here and now.* Her eyes with this kind of focus on the desired object, remind me to do the same on my desired object. Imagine the light and love we can create in our lives using this kind of Muga-mentality-focus with our heart-mind muscle empowering the focus. Our soul and spirit soar with radiance just thinking about it. Can you visualize and feel this?

Message Three

Perception is everything; it changes the thing observed and the outcome. The powerful thing you are observing right now is your current thought. Is this the future you want to call in? Put your focus on your desired way of being.

Then there is light. We hear about the speed of light and the blinding light of a world beyond. There is the brilliant strong yang light of the sun and the soothing gentle yin light of the moon. The stars have their own light. There are the colorful mysterious lights of the aurora borealis, and there is the promise of the full spectrum light of rainbows.

Look for the light throughout your day. Notice how it appears to you. Nature plays with light, especially at dawn and dusk. It dances and sparkles on water. It splashes light on the leaves of trees in the wind. The rays of the sun peek at us through the clouds. We can relate the constantly changing values of nature's light to the light of our spirit. Life is about the ebb and flow of existence. The Message shows us many ways to perceive things. Sometimes it is about seeing the space between the things. It offers us the wisdom required to anchor deep in our Inner River of Peace.

Then there is love. There are many layers and kinds of love. Our vocabulary is limited in describing them. We have the love for family, friends, home, work, and all our favorite things like heirlooms or gifts from others or gifts we give to ourselves. We love favorite times of day, hobbies, or activities. Maybe we love reading and naps. Taking a road trip, going to the movie theatre, or having coffee or tea with a friend are some of my favorite things. Little things are some of the most joyful things.

Think of times in your life when you experienced love of another kind. It made you feel differently, gave you the chills, or brought tears to your eyes. It made you pause and notice. This was a deeper beautiful kind of love that really touched your heart and soul. This is divine love. It is beyond the world of matter and form. Hold onto a time you remember this. These are moments of deep compassion, a time when love is made visible.

This love of another kind is shown to me when I see one kind of animal befriending or nursing another kind that was orphaned or injured. They create an unlikely alliance, full of nurturing and care from pure instinct. It is wonderful to see this with people. This kind of compassion for another arises from the love that is deep within us. It might be a caring touch on the shoulder, or an intuitive hug. When we receive this, we remember it.

Stop for a few moments here. Put your mind on an experience you remember that touched your heart on another level. Close your eyes, be still, and focus on how you felt during that time. Be there with your heart and mind again. With your focus amplify the feelings you had. Know you can pull up this energetic environment any time you choose. Your brain chemistry changes instantaneously to correspond with this shift in your thought, memory and feeling. These newly created chemical messengers are sent out to receptor sites on cell membranes throughout the body. This gives the cells new instructions about how to behave. Cells make up tissue; tissue makes up our physical form. Let's *Focus on the Light and Love* in our life, so this is the instructions our cells receive. Our mental and physical health depend upon it.

This self-empowering realization can be very exciting and inspiring.

Discover how it feels to be *Slow, Still, and Simple (SSS)* with the focused vision of what you want to create. Laser focus gets diluted if there are too many things involved to complicate the *real focus*. Let it be clean and clear.

What does "*and That is what You will magnify*" bring up for you?

That is the future thing your thought is creating, and *You* are the one focusing on it.

"Magnify: to intensify, to enlarge in fact or in appearance; to cause to be held in great esteem." *Webster's New World Dictionary.*

As we intensify the facts of our focus, the enlargement of them will appear. So, may our *Focus on the Light and Love* be held in great esteem.

Who among us has not played with a magnifying glass? I have childhood memories of my fascination with this. I would sit on the cement sidewalk in front of our home in Chevy Chase, Maryland, with my magnifying glass and a leaf. The magnifying glass held at just the correct angle captured the fire energy of the sun. With patience and focus, the process began: smoke appeared and a hole in the leaf started to burn.

This would not happen without all these forces coming together. The magnification of focus changed the form of the leaf, the alchemy of real focus. This kind of focus can change the thought and form of our life.

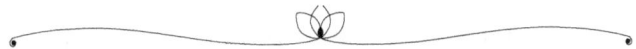

Ideas and Actions

Many times, after all these years, when I see a break in the trees with the sun rays streaming through, this Message comes back to me. Walking down our tree-covered street is one of them. The sun is a brilliant source of energy for our mind, mood, and body. Light is good medicine.

Know that you have an amazing ability to develop this kind of real focus on your personal dream-vision. The magnificent magnification of your thoughts and feelings, with clarity and continual focus will magnify. We all have a personal responsibility to be vigilant in choosing our focal points. They create our environment and our life, and they affect those around us.

Focus on the Light and Love
and That is what You will magnify.

Feel this warmth in your bones. Whether you use this message for a week or some other way, believe all the goodness and wisdom will come through at just the right instant. The longer length of time you use it, the more you will see how it shows up in many ways.

Keep this message with you. Let your heart and mind be reminded of it often. This is a magical process with a time frame of its own. Find a spot for it on your computer, phone, on an index card, or any place in your line of sight. Your car, the bathroom mirror, and your wallet are options. Keep it in a pocket close to your heart. Touch it and get it.

When we write something down, the energy moves from our heart, down our arms, and through the palms of our hands. Our hands are messengers for our hearts. Our eyes and hands work together also. Artists are experts at the ability to have their hands express what their eyes see. Writing and art are creative activities that express our heart and mind's eye through our hands. Carpenters and those creating with their hands come to mind also. Light and love are key elements of creativity. Writing The Message in a journal or on a card starts this creative process. Be your own artist of your life.

As you anchor the wisdom and love within The Message from your mental level to the cellular level, a new *holy habit* is forming. Bring The Message into your reality and trust what it offers.

This is a personal, meaningful process. Find ways that work for you and ask to be shown your way. Experiment and explore with some new ideas. Shake your existing programmed mental habits up a bit. Just by thinking a different way, our brain fires up new connections. Our perceptions change, and new windows to our soul open up. "Aha" moments are Inner River of Peace moments.

Find a *Slow, Still, and Simple (SSS)* way to keep The Message with you, day and night.

Read through the chapter, *The Power of the 5 Senses Plus 2*. Select one idea to apply to this message. Choose one you love or try a new one that rouses your curiosity. Sometimes, we just need to do something differently.

> *Example:* Focus on this message when listening to some classical or favorite inspirational music.

Message Three

Essential oil example: Peppermint (*Mentha piperita*) with its menthol zap to the brain is excellent for focus, *only if* you really love the aroma. Simply take 3-5 deep breaths from a bottle of pure peppermint, while saying The Message. Rosemary (*Rosemarinus officinalis*) is an option for mental focus.

As you focus on thinking with the heart and feeling with the mind, you tap into the powerful connection your soul and spirit have with *your* Inner River of Peace. They are an extension of each other. Cherish this way of navigating through your life. You have nothing to lose but maybe some struggle and frustration.

Focus on the Light and Love

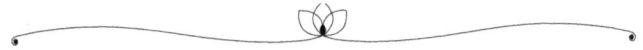

Contemplative Moments

Three Steps of Vision-Making

Engage your heart-mind muscle while sensing with your vision.

1. Set your intention-prayer with The Message and **ask** for its wisdom.
2. **Focus** on it as often as you can with your heart-mind muscle combined with a sensory action from the chapter, *The Power of the 5 Senses Plus 2*.
3. Ease up on your mental chatter trying to figure it all out. **Move** your focus to The Messenger, while doing steps 1 and 2. Be open to receiving the abundance of something better than you imagined.

Three-Step Prayer

Repeat anytime to enhance The Message.

1. Dear God, increase my awareness to receive your **Guidance.**
2. Then give me the **Courage** to follow it when I get it.
3. May I do it with the **Faith** that moves mountains - leaving no room for worries.

Message Three

Simple Focused-Breathing Technique

Do this often, anywhere.

1. **Breathe in** through your nose, while saying, **I am Focusing on the Light and Love.**

    Pause and be still.

2. **Breathe out** through your mouth, while saying, **and That is what I am magnifying.**

    Pause and be still again.

3. Do three sets of this breath experience. Each round takes about twelve seconds.

    Can you spare thirty-six seconds right now? Doing just one breath is still good.

Embrace the glimpses of wisdom, insight, and inspiration you receive from the magnificent ability to magnify where you choose to put your focus. Trusting God is part of my daily intention. It's a lifelong goal. Life is a challenging adventure. It's a smoother trip when we are connected to our Inner River of Peace.

As we increasingly master our perceptions, beliefs, and thought/feeling patterns, we magnetically attract that which we most desire.
Luanne Oakes

Try putting your focus of light and love on your desire to magnetically attract the connection to *your* Inner River of Peace. This magnifies the powerful source of great esteem that is within us, around us, and waiting to help out.

Example: I *Focus on the Light and Love* of my connection to my Inner River of Peace, *and That is what I magnify.*

Be curious and see what happens to your thinking, doing, and being. This is an adventure of the heart and mind working and playing together. Our call is to be full-of-thanks every chance we get.

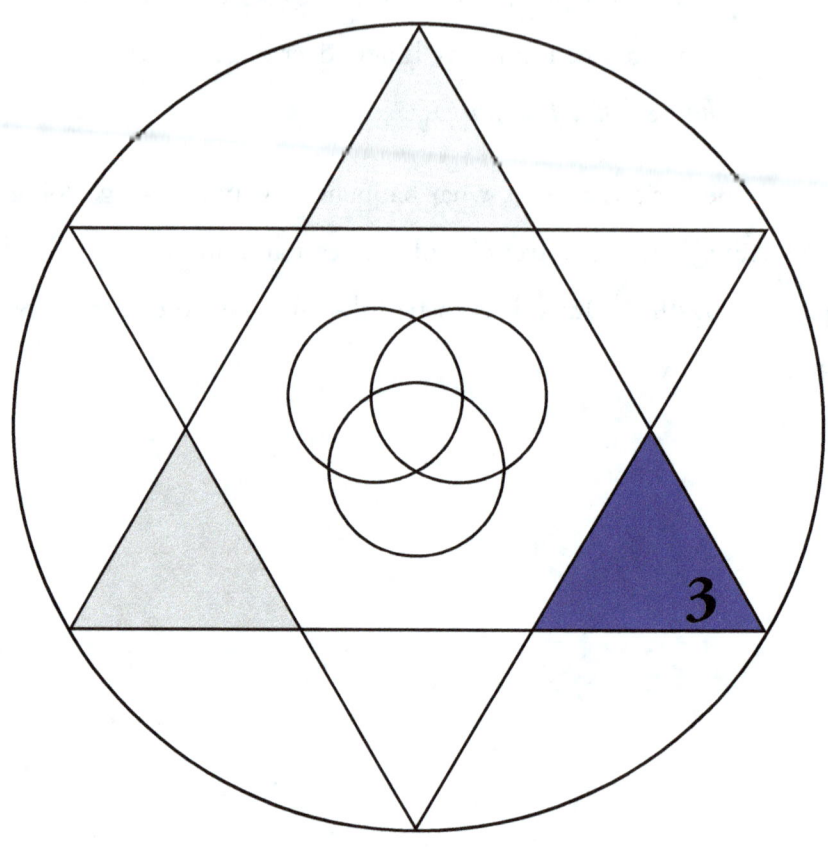

Message Three:

*Focus on the Light and Love
and That is what You will magnify.*

REVIEW
MESSAGES 1-3

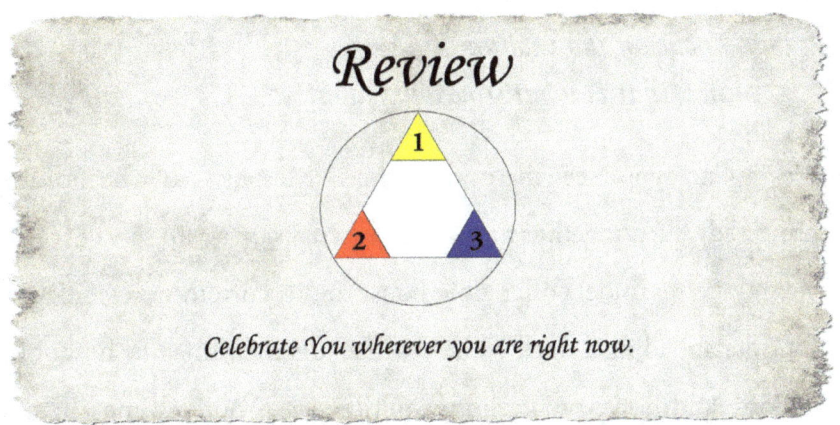

It's time to *Stop, Look, and Listen (SLL)*. This theme serves us throughout life in many situations.

What has happened so far for you with the first three Messages?

Slow down to really look at the words in each Message. Be still and reflect on the unique wisdom The Messenger offers you. It is yours for the asking. All you have to do is use the Simple Focused-Breathing Technique described at the end of each Message chapter.

Take one to three breaths with each Message below.

Review

What are you fretting about? Don't you remember?
All YOU agreed to do is:
Show Up and Hold the Vision.
We can do all the rest through you.

Whenever you Think you are limited,
Look at the sky.

Focus on the Light and Love
and That is what You will magnify.

Can you see these first three Messages are beautifully connected? Used together they create a sacred synergy to serve us well. These three reminders offer a big boost to our current state of affairs. Consider spending a week with the three together. Imagine how your thinking and how your feeling would evolve. Your cell membranes will be happy, too. Allow yourself to be inspired with this possibility.

So, how do you want to move on from here? Do you have any ideas and changes you want to make in the *holy habits* you are using to keep The Messages with you each day? As Pooh Bear says, "*Today is my favorite day!*" Making the best we can of each day, is all there really is.

Remember to create as much ease with your *holy habits* as possible, in a world of complexity and noise. Stand in your integrity with a big dose of trust and keep saddling up each day. Love, honor, and support who you really are—the very best you can. Trees are stellar examples of how to stand in integrity. The Messenger awaits to support, guide, and love us.

Review

If I Were a Tree

If I were a tree connected to thee,
you would be my ground and my sky.

My roots anchor deep in the soil of your soul,
the rock of my salvation.
My branches reach high with your Holy Spirit,
the wind of all creation.

I bathe in your moonlight of contemplation
and bask in the power and glory of your sun.
Seeing your face in my reflection
reminds me the tree and thee are truly one.

You anoint my leaves with your sacred waters
and protect me with your rainbows of grace.

Your streams at my feet sustain me
and you bring me each season to embrace.

If I were a tree connected to thee,
you would be my ground and my sky.

Whatever the season
I will dwell in your house forever,
living in the shelter of the Most High.

Candace Jean Newman

A tree teaches us about the strength, support, and nutrition that is provided as part of the natural order of existence. By anchoring deep in the roots, and reaching high with the branches and leaves, the unlimited field of possibilities meets all needs.

Thus, from an anthroposophical perspective, we anchor our physical body to the ground through and with our root chakra at the base of our spine. We connect our nonphysical spirit to the Higher Power through and with our crown chakra at the top of our head. Here we unite our scattered parts as a microcosm of the harmony created by heaven and earth. A tree is a conduit for this union.

As we open our eyes and our hearts to the trees around us, we see them in a different light. Here we remember the practice of holding a reverence for life in all things, great and small.

One of my favorite things: I love trees. When I was going for a walk in Pelican Bay in Naples, Florida, I came across a tree on the edge of a small lake. Lining my spine up with the tree, I leaned up against the trunk, glanced down at the water, and looked up at the sky. Then I sat down and wrote this poem. When my husband and I moved to the forest in Colorado, leaning up against the Ponderosa pines was one of my regular *holy habits*. Consider this: when and if a certain tree calls you over to its spot, lean into the tree, spine to

Review

trunk, and rest there. Look up at the light coming through branches and *Look at the Sky*. Ahh…

> *One touch of Nature makes the whole world kin.*
> *William Shakespeare*

As we bring our scattered parts back together in our Inner River of Peace, we are able to unite with this in others. Finally, we remember to reconnect and honor Nature, holding a reverence of life in all things great and small.

Review

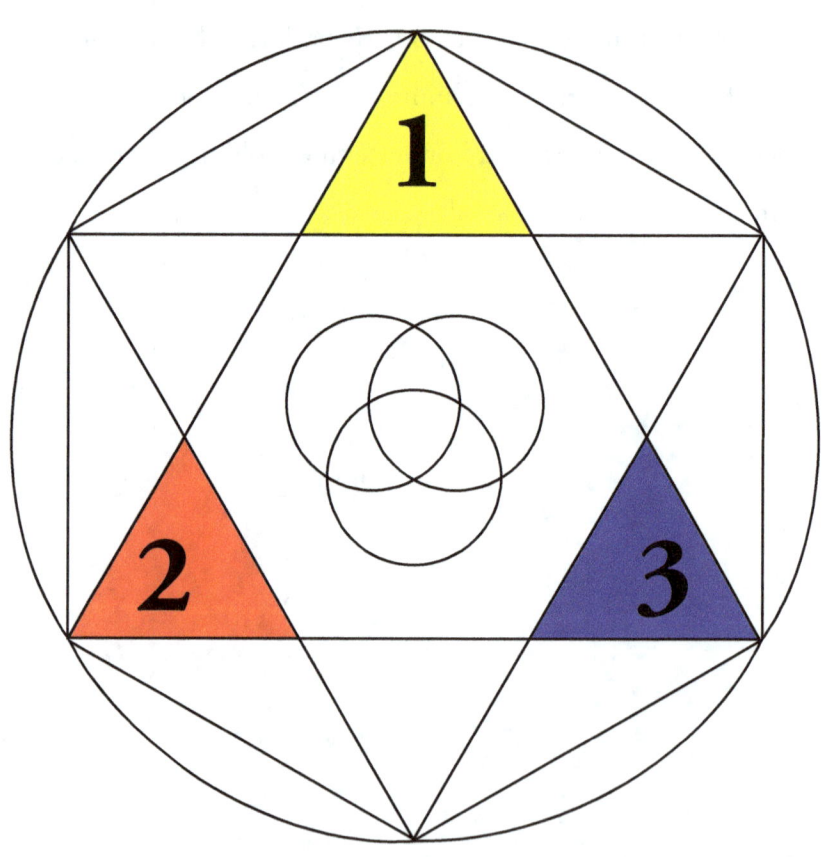

Message Four
Anchor Way Down Deep

The Message
*Anchor way down deep
in the bottom of the ocean,
and ride the waves.
Everything is OK.*

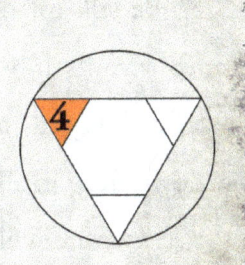

In other words, sink into the stillness that is deep inside of you where the Inner River of Peace resides. From here, simply *Stop, Look, and Listen (SLL)*. Breathe slowly and observe the waves of activity. When we are anchored in the deep calmness, we are able to observe the waves rather than be tossed in the turmoil and cacophony of the moment. From here, we are able to consciously move forward.

Notice the waves of your life events, including the thoughts and emotions that connect to them. You have now acknowledged them and named them. So, let them carry on as waves do and go by. They have a momentum of their own which eventually dissipates on its own. We don't want to hang onto them with a mighty grip and try to force the waves to go a different way. Like the tides, everything comes and goes on its own accord, eventually. On some level it is okay and will continue to be okay, somehow. Handling the waves in our life is an ongoing life process. Thank goodness for our Inner River of Peace.

Be still for one breath right now. You are already starting to anchor yourself because you are still reading. Let it happen. This powerful ability to anchor in stillness is in the core of YOU. Anchor way down deep in all the goodness you are.

If we are willing to hold the focus and wait while keeping The Message around us, the wisdom will come through when the time is right. This is not easy and its usually not a magic bullet that comes in when we want it. As we live with The Message, the power of The Messenger is available to us. The more we recognize the wisdom and give thanks, the more abundant it becomes. As we ask for and believe in this wisdom, our heart and mind continue to work together. The timing of the answer is one of the big waiting-tests of being human. The more we do this, the more we develop our patience and faith in our ability to trust the process. This is part of *Showing Up* and *Focusing on the Light and Love* of who we are.

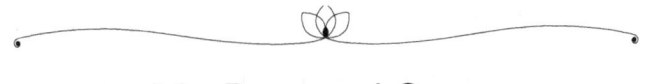

My Personal Story

Often the most trying times in our lives are when we have several big challenges going on at once. They seem to come from all directions, and we question our ability to hang on. This is a big time to anchor deeply.

One of these times for me was when my first marriage had ended, and I was living alone for the first time in my life. Being an entrepreneur by nature, I was also starting up my own business. I had just moved my aromatherapy practice from my home to a location by the city docks in Naples, Florida. This area was a spot by the water I always loved and visited often for lunch or a rest in my real estate career. Watching the lights sparkle through the trees and dance on the water and looking up at the sky was a *holy habit* of mine for years.

Moving from my home into the shop created another set of responsibilities as owner of Oil Lady Aromatherapy®. This meant running a business again and caring for my staff, handling inventory, selling, shipping, teaching, and writing. My dad called this the "whole ball of wax."

During this time, my dad's Alzheimer's had advanced to the stage where Mom and I had to place him in an Alzheimer's unit.

We had been through several years of trips to the ER with him and getting help at home for Mom. The ER doctor finally pulled us aside and said for Dad's safety and ours, it was time to take that painful leap. Within several weeks, we had Dad settled in an Alzheimer's place. A wrenching heart with lots of tears and hugs go along with this process.

Needless to say, these challenges were plenty. Along with all the above, my health was out of sorts with thyroid swings and adrenal exhaustion. There was no easy fix or overnight relief in sight. This is life's real-time evidence that stress effects our health on all levels. Stress knows no limits on our mental, emotional, physical, and spiritual health. Human beings are quite the amazing package in tough, delicate, and beautiful ways.

One night my mother called from her condo and said she wasn't feeling well. Her head was hurting, and she was very confused and unsteady. We were off to the ER at the Naples hospital, where we sat for hours while they examined her and did lots of tests. Finally, at about 5:00 a.m. in the morning, they put her in a room. I remember sitting in a chair in the corner all wrapped up in a blanket looking around at this cold, dark room. Tired and hungry, I looked over at my mother laying there quietly with her eyes closed. I prayed she was peacefully sleeping and was going to be alright.

My conversation-prayer with God went like this:

Dear God, I have a father in the Alzheimer's home whom I need to visit, a mother in the hospital bed next to me and I don't know if she's Okay or not, a shop that needs to open at 10:00am this morning, I'm bone tired, hungry and weary, and it's freezing in this room. Whatever you do, don't leave me now.

Of course, the big joke is, who's leaving whom in these times when we feel overrun with life and wiped out beyond exhaustion? We feel alone as we are trying to do what looks and feels like the impossible.

Then came The Messenger out of nowhere on a gentle wave of peace that felt like a holy warm comforter in this cold, dark room.

Anchor way down deep
in the bottom of the ocean,
and ride the waves.
Everything is OK.

The wave of peace carrying in The Message washed a stillness through me. I sat there with this strange, new feeling that not only is everything okay, but no matter what happens to Dad, Mom, me, or the shop, it's still going to be okay. This was a gentle yet powerful shift that happened in a matter of moments. In the dark sustained by the stillness, I knew it was the truth. Whatever the outcome, I would be able to handle it and be okay. I felt supported by this presence.

Message Four

I wanted to hang onto this feeling forever. It was a power that made everything okay in a mysterious way. The tired, weary, hungry self melted away. I sat there in awe and waited for Mom to open her eyes. I learned she had a mini stroke and would stay here for observation, but expected I could take her home soon. I lived most of that day in a mellow energy field that felt like a state of prayer. It was a spiritual form of nutrition that sustained me.

Getting moments and glimpses of the wisdom and spirit in these Messages give us the ability to hang on during the tough times. There are dry times and fruitful times. Once we experience the grace of the Inner River of Peace, we know it's there. We yearn for more. There is another level of thankfulness in the realization this exists. It takes courage with a big dose of trust to get through the challenges. However, we now know it's possible to experience the amazingly glorious grace of the divine spirit that sustains us.

I wouldn't begin or even try to know or explain how this happens. I do know that asking with all my heart, praying for help, and believing in the possibility adds to making it real. There is an unlimited omnipresent supply of wisdom and love for us. The sense of the sacred that came in that early morning created and sustained my new way of being for hours. So, again my trust got stronger.

It's good to be in awe of the mystery and beauty. No need to ruin or dilute it by trying to analyze it to death, dissect it to pieces, and figure it out ad nauseum. Bathing in the goodness and wisdom is the way to get the most out of it. When it comes in, ride with it. Being full-of-thanks magnifies its effect. The positive vibrations of a thankful heart attract more of its like kind.

This is science and art playing their finest symphony together. An example is Einstein's quote at the end of Message One and is worth repeating here.

The most beautiful thing we can experience is the mysterious.
It is the source of all true art and science.
Albert Einstein

Perhaps this is the Inspirational key to opening the doors to our Intuition and Imagination. These three big "I" words keep us going in the right direction. They lead us to the next big "I", as we are busy Inventing our own life.

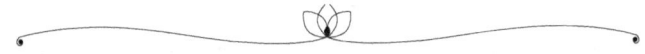

Interpretation

What does the word "Anchor" bring up to you?

Webster's New World Dictionary says, anchor is "something that serves to hold an object firmly."

Wikipedia states: "An anchor is a device, normally made of metal, used to connect a vessel to the bed of a body of water to prevent the craft from drifting due to wind or current."

How about this: The Messenger is the anchor that connects the vessel (us) to a body of water (our Inner River of Peace). This anchor prevents the craft (us again) from drifting due to the winds and currents (the waves and storms of our lives).

What does the word anchor bring up for you? Are there thoughts of a heavy energy holding you back or down? Or does it feel like a beautiful higher power that keeps you on course?

In the physical form, there are wonderful people, places, and things that provide comforting support through the ups and downs of life. On the other hand, maybe you have a strong, loving foundation of thoughts and beliefs that help anchor you. Having some of each is a worthy accomplishment in life.

An anchor holds us firmly in a particular place. It serves as a principle support or mainstay for our center of equilibrium. An anchor gives us strength and makes us feel protected and safe. It is a rock in our psyche, too. Our Inner River of Peace is an anchor holding us in a place of love and compassion. This is available to us anytime, anywhere. It flows through us.

See The Message's wisdom and love being offered to all of us, each in our own language. Its royal mission is to keep us on course, delivering the unique insights we want and need, just in the nick of time when they are most needed. Dwelling here in The Message's *shelter of the Most High* is grace. We are offered a place to rest and restore in the *shadow of the Almighty* (Psalms 91). Who among us would not want to be wrapped in the protection and love of big Angel wings?

What does *"way down deep in the bottom of the ocean"* mean to you?

There is an ocean of courage and love way down deep within us, and it is inexhaustible. We are part of the oceanic-type field of the universe. We forget or ignore this because we get focused on the daily doings and demands of our physical life. The challenges of life, with all its worries and fears, can drain our precious life force energy *if* we let it. The wild monkeys of the mind like to keep us distracted and very busy. Sometimes, it gets pretty wild up there with all the chatter. There are times I feel like the crazy monkeys called in a convention. It's time to go slow, still the mind, and return to the simple Message.

The Messages offer us a ray of light and help us disengage. When we *Stop, Look, and Listen (SLL)* for a few moments in time, we open ourselves up by creating space for the arrival of the love and wisdom. Wisdom is waiting to be invited in. Because the wisdom is personal, The Message touches our heart and spirit on an intimate level. Sometimes, it seems like its waiting on the other side of the door. Knock, wait, and it shall open.

All you need to do is keep The Message with you. Just think about it and hold it dearly in your heart. Open hands and open hearts create open minds. It is also true the other way around. Compassion comes forth.

The Messages remind us that it's okay to take a break from the nonsense of the world. It's a real treat sometimes to give our whole self a chance to consciously breathe. Break-away moments of disengagement are whatever you can manage to do at the time. It can be walking outside and looking at the sky, meditating, sitting by a tree at the end of your day on the way home, or going to a monastery for a few hours or days. A library is a favorite place of mine for quiet and time-out. Maybe it's just pausing a few moments to gaze out the window. Even if it's only sitting at the stop light and looking at the sky, it counts.

Remember the value of day-dreaming that so many geniuses value. Give your genius element some time and attention. What we feed, and what we nurture is what grows within us. There are so many options for ways to pause. This is a time again to be *Slow, Still, and Simple (SSS)*.

I just did this right now while typing this section of the book. I stopped and looked out at the ocean with its beautiful waves rolling in just outside the condo window in New Smyrna Beach, Florida. I got still and listened. I heard: *"How wonderful. You're starting to get more balance with your type-A personality work pattern. Keep this up, do what you love with discernment, and you won't have to burn out again."*

I send this vision-memory of the ocean to inspire you to pause here, too. If you don't have an ocean memory, use your imagination. There is no reason we can't find these moments of personal treasure in our heart and mind. Love *your* Inner River of Peace as it flows with ease deep within your heart.

Going *way down deep in the bottom of the ocean* is a call to be true to our heart and soul. It asks that we take the pauses and the breaks that we need. This is not a selfish thing as many like to think. It's actually a self-full thing. We are a more fulfilled person when we feel well, and then we have this to give to others. As a bit of a workaholic on some kind of mission most of my life, I know it takes continual effort and time to really stay in tune with all our scattered parts. Treating myself to massages and taking naps didn't happen until after my first burnout. God willing and the creek don't rise, I'm getting better at this all the time.

Go through your life this week or maybe even longer with this Message way down deep within your heart. Imagine how you can feel with this part of you functioning so well. Pull up a memory of a time you experienced this. Tapping into your inspirational well in the oasis of life, brings back the feeling of being fully alive again. Return to this vision as often as you can. Anchoring deep in *your* Inner River of Peace is a moment-by-moment thing. It is possible for sure.

What do "*waves*" mean to you?
How can some of these waves possibly be okay?

Webster's New World Dictionary describes waves as: "a disturbance or variation that transfers energy progressively from point to point in a medium. A moving ridge or swell on the surface of a liquid (as of the sea); something that swells and dies away; a surge of sensation or emotion such as a wave of anger swept over her."

We all know about the waves in oceans that dissipate as they come on shore. There are waves and swings of our emotions, too. Emotions come and go like waves and the winds of change. These experiences are part of the circle of life. This is all the more reason to be anchored in our Inner River of Peace. So, going way down below the tumultuous waves is the place to be. Scuba divers experience this. My husband tells me of the quiet peace of going deep and the sound of his breath there. He also tells me of this same experience when he was flying his airplane above the clouds. We can become a calm center in the swirling circle of activity.

Anchor Way Down Deep

Waves are constantly in motion: coming and going, rolling and crashing, forming and dissipating. This certainly sounds like lots of events in life. There are the waves of each day, and the waves of each season of life. Some waves last a lifetime. Life brings in waves of all kinds. They can be about health, family, relationships, jobs, and money. Waves bring up emotions such as fear, worries, doubts, regrets of the past, and concerns of the future. There are also waves of peace and waves of love to be cherished. Thank goodness for the ebb and the flow.

Sometimes waves come in and we wonder how they could possibly be okay. How can we find any peace or a way to resolve this wave? The all-powerful source of strength within each of us is rarely experienced. We don't know it's there until we experience it. We think we can't handle something. The trust in our ability to endure or resolve it gets questioned.

Anchor way down deep
in the bottom of the ocean,
and ride the waves.
Everything is OK.

Whether the waves are small rises or towering tsunamis, they will pass or evolve into something else. Nature shows us this. Each wave continues to make us who we are. The stronger our anchor is in our Inner River of Peace, the stronger our heart-mind muscle becomes. We become better and more prepared to handle the next wave.

Discover the beauty of tapping into the source of strength that awaits our call. The possibilities are unknown until we walk the path with a sense of hope and wonder. Look at what it takes for a plant to produce a flower. It all starts with a tiny seed that needs to be nurtured to grow into its highest Self. The act of creation is amazing. Be curious about how The Message can embrace and nurture you.

Ideas and Actions

Record The Message in the most convenient place for you. Keep it simple. Try observing how your heart can think and your mind can feel. Many of The Messages on my index cards have different months and years listed by them. It reminds me how they have delivered wisdom to me again and again over the years. There are no expiration dates on universal truths of love.

Real truths are always real. Real wisdom is always there. Real love is found here.

Anchor Way Down Deep

I am *Showing Up and Holding the Vision* with this book for you to create your way for The Message to become a part of your life. This happens through osmosis if we do it often enough. *Holy habits* are great habits that enrich and change our lives. Explore and experiment with a way that is meaningful to you, and full of love.

You don't have to be a writer to record your message. Keep it on your refrigerator, computer desktop, phone, or another device. Your breakfast table, desk area, dresser, or bathroom mirror, and your credit card spot are options. Any place in your line of sight will do. Try your hip pocket or close to your heart. As you touch it, you remember it.

> *Anchor way down deep*
> *in the bottom of the ocean,*
> *and ride the waves.*
> *Everything is OK.*

As you continue to go through this book, you will come around to the best way The Messages work for you. These are powerful tools you are putting in your toolbox to continually serve you throughout life. If this were not true, I would not be writing this book.

However long you decide to use The Message, set the intention to get all the goodness and wisdom it offers. The longer length of time you use it, the more you will see how many times it keeps popping up to serve you well. It becomes part of the autonomic nervous system response. This anchors the wisdom from your mental plane into your body on the cellular level. As your mind shifts, your physical chemistry changes. A new *holy habit* is forming in your energy field, too.

Ask The Messenger to show you what you need to know to take your next step. The Message is the spark that brings forth the golden nuggets waiting for you to discover. The wisdom and love come from another place and expands your horizons.

Choose *Slow, Still, and Simple (SSS)* ways that enrich your life.

Read through the chapter, *The Power of the 5 Senses Plus 2*. Select one idea to apply to this message. Choose one you love or try a new one that rouses your curiosity. Sometimes, we just need to try something new to fire-up new neurons in the brain and the heart.

> *Example:* Anchor in this message while dancing or moving around to your favorite music. Think of The Message while doing yoga or tai chi.
>
> *Essential oil example*: Sandalwood (*Santalum album*) or patchouli (*Pogostemon cablin*) are some of the best essential oils for anchoring. They offer deep, rich, and grounding aromas through their thick viscous liquids. Be

sure you love the aroma you choose. As often as you like take 3-5 deep breaths from the bottle of pure essential oil. Close your eyes and imagine anchoring The Message in your brain's limbic system.

Message Four

Contemplative Moments

Three Steps of Vision-Making

Engage your heart-mind muscle while sensing with your vision.

1. Set your desire and prayer with The Message and **ask** to be shown its wisdom.
2. **Anchor** it daily with your heart-mind muscle combined with a sensory action. See the chapter, *The Power of the 5 Senses Plus 2.*
3. Release your tight thoughts trying to MAKE what you *think* should happen. Believe you are **open** to receive the abundance as you release your mind from its box of preconceived thoughts and feelings. Use your Imagination to help you do this. The abundance and wisdom that comes in may be way beyond what you *think* is possible.

Three-Step Prayer

Repeat anytime to enhance The Message.

1. Dear God, increase my awareness to receive your **Guidance.**
2. Then give me the **Courage** to follow it when I get it.
3. May I do it with a **Faith** that can move mountains, leaving no room for worries.

Anchor Way Down Deep

Simple Focused-Breathing Technique

Do this often, anywhere.

1. **Breathe in** through your nose, while saying**, I am Anchoring way down deep in the bottom of the ocean.**

    Pause and be Still.

2. **Breathe out** through your mouth, while saying, **I am riding the waves, and I know I'm OK.**

    Pause and be still again.

3. Do three sets of this breath experience now. Each round takes about twelve seconds.

    Can you spare thirty-six seconds right now to try this?

Life is a challenging adventure. It's a smoother trip when we have the tools to anchor in our Inner River of Peace. The tools are weightless and don't take up any space. As with all tools, they are happiest being used regularly to serve you with the heart and mind's desires.

Only by searching and mining are gold and diamonds obtained, and
man can find every truth connected with his being,
if he will dig deep into the mine of his soul.
James Allen, *As a Man Thinketh*

So, let's go searching for the gold (the wisdom) and find the truth (The Messenger) that is connected to our being, as we dive

Message Four

deep into the mine of our soul (as we anchor deep in our Inner River of Peace).

Sometimes, I think of life as a big expedition to explore each part of our path and ride the waves to find the treasures of wisdom and grace. These hidden treasures are always within us somewhere. The heart of the explorer in us all gives us courage and inspiration to continue the exploration for these gemstones that take us to our Inner River of Peace.

May the results of bringing this Message into your life give you a feeling of liberation, a freedom from feeling tossed around in the turbulent waves of life. Waves go by and the sun rises at some point in time. We know there is always nighttime and there is always daytime. With a foot in each world, we carry on.

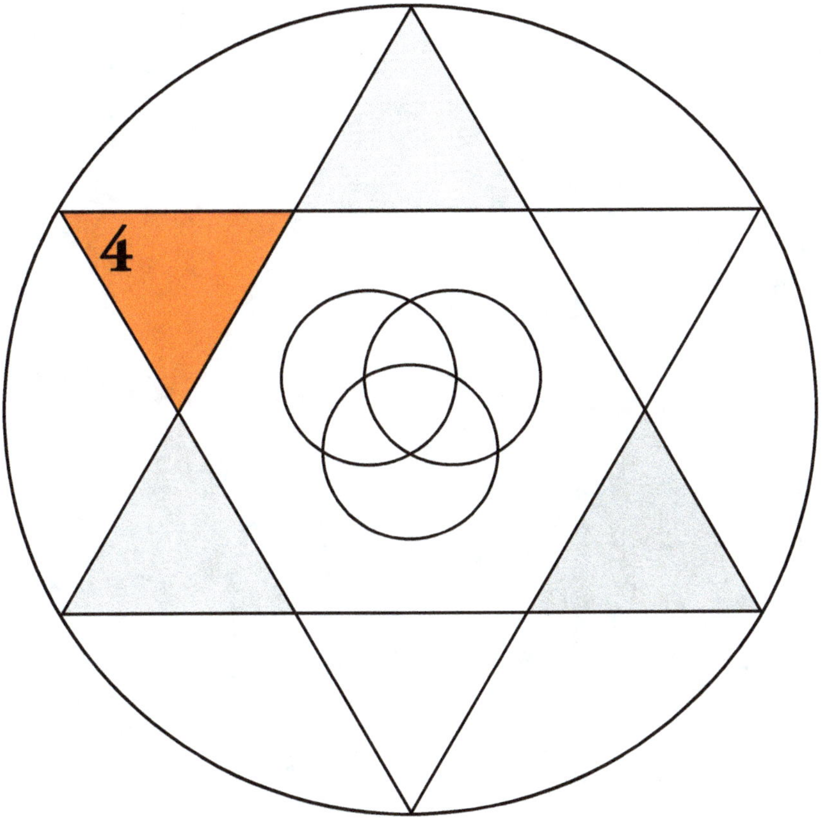

Message Four:

*Anchor way down deep
in the bottom of the ocean,
and ride the waves.
Everything is OK.*

Message Five
Keep Me with You

The Message

*Keep Me with You,
just Keep Me with You.*

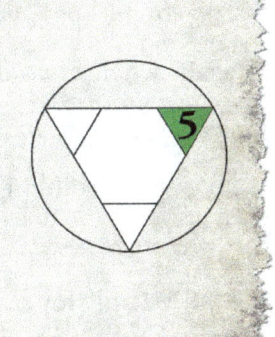

In other words, no matter what is going on, stay connected to The Messenger. We know one of the absolutes in life is that things change. The Messenger comes as a Great Comforter to remind us we are not alone. You may be going through something tough, and it may get tougher. It might be an exciting new shift. You might sense a transition of some sort is in the works. These are words of comfort, love, and support. Whether it's a tough change, an exciting event, or ordinary daily events, The Messenger is there with these words: just *Keep Me with You.*

Message Five

The first time I received this Message, it seemed The Messenger was saying: *If you don't keep me with you and decide to go it alone, then I can't get the love and wisdom to you that is always here. Things are a lot tougher when you do it by yourself. I am here, and I'm not leaving you. So, come unto me, rest with me, and don't let go of my hand.*

In the past year of writing this book, The Message came in again when I was doubting myself. Following it I heard, *I've got your back, and all the rest of you, too.* I smiled and kept on writing. I smile again, thinking about what The Messenger has for you with this Message.

Be still for one breath here. Reflect what it would be like to know you don't have to handle things by yourself. What a comforting idea. Hold on to this thought and feeling. Now we are talking about trust again. Trusting our self to not hold our fists so tightly that water can't even get in.

Trusting The Messenger to be there for us changes our life. Possibilities of all kinds are available when we choose to trust. We become a more radiant being. Haven't we already learned or sensed this is possible? Why would we choose otherwise?

Your Inner River of Peace awaits your decision. These are soulful times.

Keep Me with You

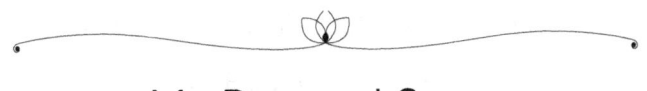

My Personal Story

One particular early morning, I was suddenly awakened from a deep sleep at 4:00 a.m. This happens to be the time I was born in the mountains in Pittsfield, Massachusetts. Throughout my life, many of The Messages and other words of wisdom come in around 4:00 a.m. I sat straight up in bed, and in came the wave of peace with its companion of stillness:

*Keep Me with You,
just Keep Me with You.*

It was short, sweet, clear, and succinct. I paused in the stillness, reflecting upon my life at that time. There had been lots on my mind for quite a while. An extra dose of comfort and support of another kind was just what the good doctor ordered. Each Message always has its own time frame and it is brilliant. We often don't realize this until later.

I happened to be in the midst of my ten-year real estate career, and I was having a lot of pain from a weight-lifting injury doing squats. My low back got torqued and the pinched nerve came around the front of my hip and down my leg. Much later and after many doctor visits, I found out the nerve and my ovarian cyst predicament aggravated each other. The nerve pain and cyst pain together determined my lifestyle for many years until the cyst ruptured. The pain controlled my lifestyle and disrupted my sleep patterns. Sometimes, I just didn't sleep.

I had been feeling unsettled for a couple of years trying to sort this out. With over a five-year search for the cause and solution to the pain, one would think this would have been fairly easy to diagnose and resolve. There were trips to all kinds of doctors and the ER room due to a small cyst rupture that was not diagnosed, so it absorbed on its own over a few days. I visited various health centers including Kenneth Cooper's Clinic in Texas, and Hippocrates Health Institute in Florida. My symptoms and the cause were not getting resolved. Being health-minded and fit most of my life just added to my frustration. Too many things were building up, and I was wearing down. I sensed that a life shift was brewing.

When The Message came in early that morning, it confirmed my thoughts. It left me feeling I would know what I needed to know when I needed to know it. I would be shown the way at that time. Meanwhile, I needed to start building up my strength and spirit for handling whatever changes were in the wind. Events were going to change in my life, and things would be different.

Indeed, they did. The physical pain and mental-emotional fatigue forced me to leave my position with the real estate company I loved. My cyst ruptured in a cabin with no phone in the North

Keep Me with You

Carolina mountains and it was days before the big surgery. All this started a new season of my life.

This was a worthy life lesson in hindsight, of course. The whole experience took about six years. It revealed to me that when we have pain, our call is to follow it. Don't give up searching as long as there is still one viable resource left to try. We dig deep as investigators and explorers. This ruptured cyst and nerve pain did not need a rocket scientist to figure it out. However, my life lesson was about the pain it took to shift me to my life's work and called me to be more of the part of me that was demanding I acknowledge and embrace.

Without pain as the motivator, I would not have been on so many explorations for knowledge and wisdom. One of them introduced me to essential oils. A therapist from England used these precious liquids in a massage, and I felt like I had found an oasis that was saving my life. Essential oils showed me the relief I needed and paved the way to move forward with the next step in my life. They revealed the love I felt as a little girl really existed. This was in the 1980s. I was very sensitive to smells and had never heard of essential oils or the word *aromatherapy*. I share more in the chapter, *Essential Oils as Soulful Elements*.

Honoring our own unique life path and purpose is what The Messages offer. The love and support for our true self grow stronger, IF we accept this assignment and alignment. All we have to do is *Show Up and Hold the Vision.* This is all the more reason to keep developing a stronger bond with our Inner River of Peace. This is an energy cord not to be broken. It is precious. Keep it with you, just keep it with you— wherever you are.

Interpretation

What does "*Keep*" bring up for you?

"Keep: to retain in one's possession or power; to be faithful to keep a promise; to act fittingly in relation to keep the Sabbath; to conform to habits or conduct; preserve, maintain, such as to watch over and keep us from harm; to take care of." *Webster's New World Dictionary.*

A keeper is someone who watches over and cares for another. The idea of the Higher Power, watching over and caring for us is part of divine order, divine timing, and divine grace. Saying the Lord's Prayer is one way of keeping God with us. Throughout all cultures, there have been prayers and services performed to keep one connected to the Divine, and there is traditionally a giving of great thanks. It often includes aromas such as frankincense or rose, to clear the air and lift up the prayers.

Simply reflecting on The Message throughout our day brings it into our being. Once we start relating the wisdom from The Message to our current life, it becomes more meaningful. We develop a very personal relationship with The Message and The Messenger behind The Message. This only gets more amazing and beautiful as we carry on through life's adventures. Our tool bag gets lighter and more powerful.

Who is 'Me'?

'Me' is The Messenger delivering this Message. So, who is The Messenger to you? *Stop, Look, and Listen (SLL)* for a few minutes to reflect on this. You might want to go back to the beginning and take a look again at the chapter, *Who Is The Messenger?* It can offer you more insights at this point in the book. Reminisce about times in life you felt this presence around you.

What experiences in life created your belief system? Some scientists know and talk about a force, a source, and the infinite energy that operates and creates beyond our realm of understanding and power. Many want to know how God thinks. Plugging into this power source is our biggest and strongest energy cord. As we nurture and cherish this cord, it is strengthened. The power of prayer knows no distance and has no limitations. Its field of influence moves into the unknown. We can't see it, but we can believe it.

Who is 'You'?

Well, this is the other big question of the universe. There are many parts, levels, dimensions of who we actually are being. First, we have our physical body, a vessel to honor and protect, with all its various parts. It needs all kinds of care and maintenance to keep it functioning. It is a temple for our soul, and it is also a chemistry tube constantly popping and fizzling as it strives to maintain homeostasis.

The physical part of us we visually see is part of the physical world of matter and form. Therefore, our physical body demands and gets most of our attention. Life around us makes sure we get lots of news about what the body should look like and how it can be more beautiful and healthier. This is often to the detriment of our emotional state, our spiritual life, and our soul. The Messages are on a mission to bring our true and whole self into harmony. All our scattered parts yearn to dance together.

The nonphysical parts of us include our thoughts and emotions. Our emotions spontaneously create corresponding biochemicals that the brain sends to cells throughout our body. Eventually, all this is reflected in the state of our health. The spirit and the soul surround and permeate every part of us. They are always trying to get our attention. They wait. Often, they try sending us

Keep Me with You

messages in many different forms, like aches and pains. If we don't listen after a certain amount of time, we get hit with a spiritual two-by-four to get our attention. This usually involves a pretty big lesson, demanding and forcing a course correction in our life. Maybe we can learn to respond to the hint, before the two-by-four arrives. Oh, how our soul can speak to us through our body.

Our energy body is affected by our emotions, and this effects the physical body. We've all been under stress and found ourselves coming down with a very bad cold. The grief suffered from the loss of a loved one often coincides with some form of the crud or total exhaustion that puts us to bed.

Our parts are so interconnected and interdependent we are not allowed to treat them separately without effecting the whole. Some parts get ignored with the demands of the moment. The complex multi-*asking* world we live in is very demanding. Without discernment, we can really get out of whack. This is burnout. The worldly ways usually don't encourage taking breaks or thinking about keeping The Messenger with us. Practicing the presence of God calls for holding on to spirit-and-soul consciousness. We can do this with our consciously newly created *holy habits*.

In a simple and profound way may we respond to the call:

Keep Me with You,
just Keep Me with You.

Message Five

This is one of The Messages that keeps coming up the most often in my life. I realize now, it's a short simple form of prayer that applies to just about everything. It reminds me to stay close, hold hands, and trust the power of the Great Holy Spirit that surrounds and plays through us.

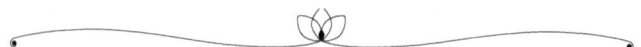

Ideas and Actions

Add this Message to your journal or other device with the date. There may be other future dates and events you want to add to it. Note a situation you are in currently, and any wisdom or insights coming through for you. Looking back on notes we've made with The Message, or having a memory come up of a time gone before, deepens our understanding later in life. This is one reason why I wrote this book. I had to relive each Message and life situation that called it in, in order to write about it.

*Keep Me with You,
just Keep Me with You.*

Keep Me with You

Read or say this short Message often and notice how it fits into your life at this time. Let it reveal more about who you are. It will let you know what you need to know, when you need to know it.

Whether you use this message for seven days or a month, or even just a day, set the intention to get all the goodness and wisdom it has for your personally. You also might notice how it can speak to others close to you. The longer length of time you use it, the more it strengthens and assists you on deeper levels throughout your life. With repeated use, it becomes part of your autonomic nervous system response to life situations.

When you move the wisdom from your mental plane into your body on the cellular level, your heart-mind muscle is energized. This new way of thinking and feeling gradually becomes a new *holy habit*. Creating a new habit takes time. Many of our old ones are deeply rooted in the core of our being. Trusting and taking action to renew our spirit in this way, increases our vitality to assist the shift. I believe the shifts are there to be made. However, we have to do our part of thinking, feeling and acting with love to open the channel.

This Message of universal truth has golden nuggets for you to discover. They reveal secret hidden treasures of wisdom and love. They arrive just when you need them most.

Message Five

Be *Slow, Still, and Simple (SSS)* in creating ways to keep The Message with you. Simply find your way that works with ease. Experiment and explore new ideas. Shake up the programmed mental process, by turning your gaze and focusing intently on new ideals that serve you well.

Read through the chapter, *The Power of the 5 Senses Plus 2*. Select an idea to combine with The Message. Change it up a bit and explore your senses with something new.

Example: Think about this message when you are gardening (maybe even with your hands in the dirt), arranging flowers or doing yard work. Hands are very expressive, and they are connected to our hearts. Take good care of them.

Essential oil example: Eucalyptus (*Eucalyptus radiata*) is a good choice to keep us on tract, *only if* you really like the aroma. It's warming and stimulating, and gets the rivers moving in the body. This is a top respiratory oil and encourages us to breathe deeply. Repeat The Message to yourself as you breathe pure Eucalyptus from the bottle into your brain and lungs. Take 3-5 breaths with the Simple Focused-

Breathing Technique at the end of *Contemplative Moments*. Ravintsara (*Cinnamomum camphora*) is another top respiratory choice. Both these essential oils are good for focus and clarity. The side effect is they boost your immune system too.

Message Five

Contemplative Moments
Three Steps of Vision-Making

Engage your heart-mind muscle while sensing with your vision.

1. Set your intention-prayer with The Message and **ask** for its wisdom for your specific situation.
2. **Keep** this Message and The Messenger with you. Let it engage your heart-mind muscle combined with a sensory action from the chapter: *The Power of the 5 Senses Plus 2*.
3. **Release** your thoughts of trying to control a certain outcome. Do this by claiming the power in The Message and seeing a different way. Acknowledge where you are and be open to trusting The Messenger.

Three-Step Prayer

Repeat anytime to enhance The Message.

1. Dear God, increase my awareness to receive your **Guidance.**
2. Then give me the **Courage** to follow it when I get it.
3. May I do it with the **Faith** that moves mountains - and not let go of your hand.

Simple Focused-Breathing Technique

Do this often, anywhere. Try holding a bottle of your favorite pure essential oil to your nose while breathing. This fires

The *Message of Love* into your brain and lungs. Receptor sites on your cells throughout your body receive these new corresponding biochemical messengers of emotion.

1. **Breathe in** through your nose, while saying, ***I am Keeping You with Me.***

    Pause and be Still.

2. **Breathe out** through your mouth, while saying, ***I am just Keeping You with Me.***

    Pause and be still again.

3. Claim the next thirty-six seconds and pause with three sets of this breathing technique. Breath The Message into the power of your heart-mind muscle with your favorite aroma. This new way of thinking and feeling creates new *holy habits* on a cellular level. Happy thoughts create happy cells.

May you experience and enjoy a form of comfort and support from this Message that sustains you. It is here to remind us we don't have to go it alone. It is here to serve us well for the asking.

This is an adventure for all the many magnificent parts of you. Anchor deep in your heart's love. The Messenger resides in our heart and all the other parts of us, patiently waiting for us to come home to our Self. Practice the prayer and intention of keeping The Messenger with you. There is peace in this practice.

Be full-of-thanks every chance you get.

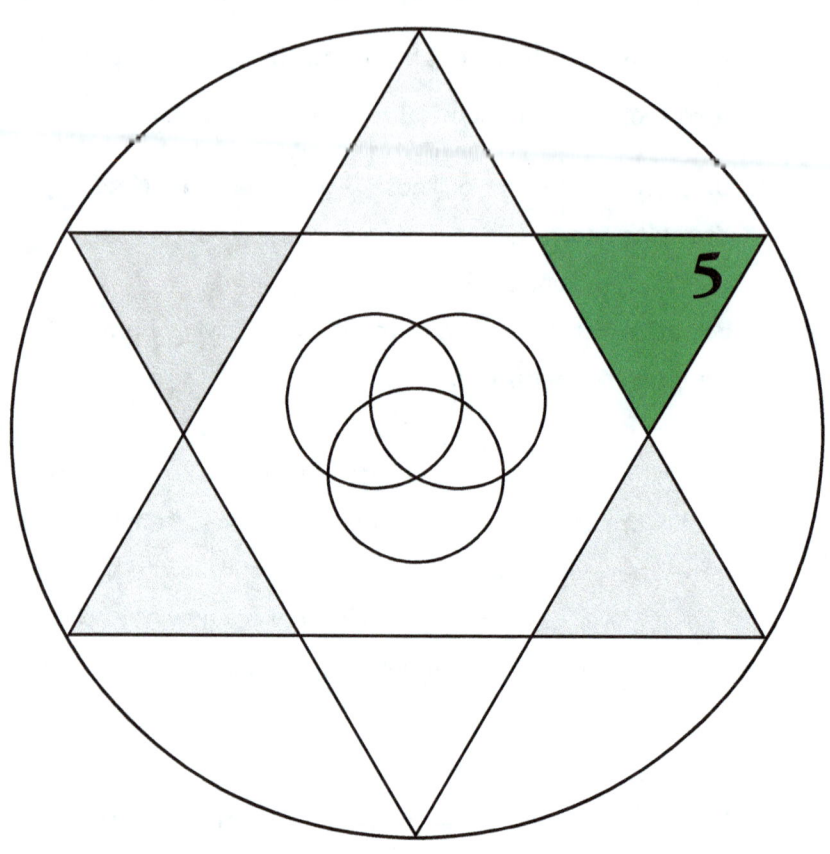

Message Five:

*Keep Me with You,
just Keep Me with You.*

Message Six
Don't Resist the Web of Life

The Message

Don't resist, pull, push, or struggle in the web of this life you're in. Everyone is in the web of life. Be there with it, in all its turmoil, and peace shall prevail.

In other words, strife is going to be part of our life, because it is part of the circle of life. Peace is also a part of the circle of life. Be who you are in it. Play your part in the web of life. All things are provided when we stop desperately trying to make what we want to happen or when we decide we can figure it out all on our own.

Instead of pulling back or pushing forward until we are completely out of sorts, let's *Stop, Look, and Listen (SLL)*. Turn around and see it, name it, and know it's here with you at this time. It's taking you somewhere. You may not know where you are going. However, be assured you are on your way. To shove it down and get more irritated, just calls in more turmoil. The cycle only gets worse. We all know this. Claim the higher road of genuine power and move into *your* Inner River of Peace.

My Personal Story

Daily life provides many opportunities to experience what this Message conveys. The ups and downs of life are cycles of resisting and releasing, struggling and flowing. The Message can also play through our dream time. Our nightly dreams show us some of the real things we are dealing with in the river of life. Struggling in dreams can be as tough as struggling in waking life. It's another way that our soul can get our attention. Sometimes, our dreams can clear something up, can answer a question, and can give us a solution for things in our waking life.

Humans have been fascinated and puzzled by dreams as long as they have been sleeping. It is a mysterious world with layers of consciousness, each delivering messages of their own. Trying to understand them is also an age-old dilemma. As long as we are here, we'll continually be living with dreams. Cycles of waking and sleeping goes with the territory. We have dreams in both parts of this

Don't Resist the Web of Life

cycle. Some of us dream a lot, and others dream very seldom. Some we remember, many we don't. Our relationship with our dreams is unique to each of us. Just recognizing them, observing how they make us feel, and listening is a tremendous insight into our lives.

My dream world is sometimes so clear and real that I wonder where the lines of the sleeping and waking world are. There are times when I feel the emotions so intensely that I awaken with my body in the same emotional and physical pain as it was in the dream state. Which is real? They are both parts of our whole self. Dreams serve a real purpose in releasing emotions, showing us what we need to know, and letting us know how we are doing. They bring up things in other levels of consciousness to get our attention.

I have learned things in my dreams that I haven't experienced in my waking life. However, the dream experience was so vivid, I seem to understand what it would be like in the waking world. Each world reflects the other in different levels of consciousness.

For this brief interlude on dreams, their power, and their wisdom, I am writing about two categories that I've experienced in many ways throughout my life. Many of our dreams are around the human issues of struggle and resistance, pushing and pulling about something. The **struggling dreams** tend to leave us anxious and tight. The **resolution dreams** provide relief and insight.

Struggling Dreams

Several of my dreams have reoccurring themes with boats and rivers. One very vivid dream was being in a boat and struggling to make it go the way I wanted it to go. The river was not in agreement with my agenda. Trying to steer a boat (me) against the current (natural rhythm of water) is a big struggle. I was paddling and straining like crazy to force the situation. Imagine what it feels like to row a boat up stream. This was exhausting and frustrating. I awakened in a tight knot. I had a sense I needed to either turn the boat around and flow with the current—or get out of the boat and get in the river. The answer is not always clear regarding what is really going on underneath the boat and in the current.

There have also been dreams when I couldn't get my legs to run. I wanted so badly to move forward faster. No matter how hard I focused and tried to get them to run, even trying to pick up my legs, I could not make it happen. This dream theme also came through trying to control a car. The pedals to go fast or stop were not responding. Sometimes my eyes would close, and I could not get them open to see if the car was on the road. Plenty of frustration and struggle was going on here.

All these struggle dreams indicate not going with the flow of life at the time. I needed to ease up on my own agenda for what I thought was the way. I needed to initiate ways to release the struggle that was taking me down. If we pause and recognize the rough spots in life for what they are, we can start to ease up on the pushing and pulling. They clear up in time and with lots of prayer. Then, we can chart a peaceful course with renewed wisdom and insights, which gives us a new course with new ways to travel our river of life.

Making the decision to wait for clearer wisdom is also a form of action. The power of our words plays in here. Using different words is a form of good nutrition for the heart and mind. This helps us know what to do and how to be. It affects those around us and helps shift the stressful situation. Drop by drop on the smooth waters of an enlightened decision, a ring of peace is created.

When the struggle is great and seems to go on forever with no resolution no matter how hard we try, we awaken feeling drained. Even though dreams are only part of the night's sleep, it can feel like the whole night. Restful sleep eludes us.

Struggle dreams are often about getting in line with our purpose, our call, our mission in life. This is a heart, mind, and soul journey. These are lifetime questions and require climbing our mountains, one sacred step at a time. Part of the answer is to become quiet with our Inner River of Peace. The Message lovingly embraces our parts to take us there. Be still, step aside and observe for a while. In quietness comes great strength. Ask yourself what is *really* going on?

Message Six

Resolution Dreams

I love animals. They are such a gift and teach us important things like loyalty and love. My only pets have been dogs, and they taught me all about loyalty and love. According to Native American teachings, this is their animal medicine for us humans. We are either in balance with loyalty and love, or out of sorts with it. There is a good and not-so-good part of everything in this world of duality. We want to watch for the tipping point.

When we lived in Colorado, it was a thrill to watch the deer, elk, and horses. At the beach in Florida, the birds and dolphins are some of the teachers. I love to walk down our street in the Mt. Dora area of Florida and visit the horses, cows, and donkeys along the way. Sometimes, they come over to the fence, and I can love on them. My dreams have provided many profound experiences with animals. Some of them have been so vivid, that in waking life I seem to understand them. I am beyond grateful for this. When I see a whale or a horse, I feel like I know them because of these two dreams.

In the whale dream, I was out on a raft in the Gulf of Mexico in Naples, Florida, and fell asleep. Suddenly awakening, I found myself way out beyond the Naples Pier. Panic and fear set in because I didn't know how I'd get all the way back to shore. I'm lying face down on the raft and paddling as hard as I can, getting nowhere fast. Suddenly, I felt this huge surge beneath me that was slowly moving me back toward shore. Fear set in, I paddled harder and was afraid to look and see what it was. Finally, the fear got so great, I turned my head to see what was there. Right behind me was a huge back barely breaking the surface. It was much bigger than my raft. I could feel this massive power underneath me that was much greater than me. After more minutes of shear fright, I started to breath with the whale and the swells. Instantaneously, I become eerily calm. An amber glow surrounded us. There was no more paddling. As I breathed with the whale, I glided with ease into shore. The relief was effortless and has become a profound memory for trusting in the loving power that is stronger than any of us. The breath is the connector, the portal, to this power of peace.

In the horse dream, I was in a big open field with a beautiful chestnut horse. When I was walking in the field, my legs were very heavy and so was my spirit. It was a big struggle to lift each leg. Then, I got on the bare back of the horse, we galloped across the fields with no effort at all. Nothing hurt in my body at all and the heaviness lifted immediately. I tried walking and riding a couple of times in the dream with the same results. Riding the horse was like the effortless spirit of the wind. It felt like the horse and I were one since all the struggling had released. We laid down in the grass together to rest. The left side of my face laid flat on the horse's big flat right cheek. I started breathing in his cadence. His big nostrils had a sweet sound and soft smell. As long as I stayed there in rhythm with his breath, my burdens of struggle subsided. I was in the flow of Great Spirit. The oneness of grace prevailed. When I stayed in the drudgery of the land (struggles) of life, I was heavy and out of balance. When I connected to my spirit and soul (represented by the horse), I still covered the ground; however, it was with ease and flow. It is a constantly moving target to keep all our parts in harmony. We find our Inner River of Peace when we do. The Messages offer again to be one way of wisdom and love that takes us there. The Messenger is magnificent.

Each animal instinctively taught me to quietly breathe with the situation and follow my gut instinct. When you know something is genuine, you simply know it. There is no pro-con list or need to analyze it to smithereens. There was extreme doubt and fear in each dream. As soon as I thought I couldn't handle this painful fear another second, something made me turn around, face it, and embrace the animal with my breathing. When I started this breathing with the animal's natural rhythm, in came an amazing sense of harmony and oneness. Any kind of stress or fear in the dream simply melted away. The cadence of our breathing can release fear, and our thoughts and emotions shift. The Inner River of Peace prevails.

Don't Resist the Web of Life

Animals carry their own wisdom-medicine. This is an intricate part of life for indigenous peoples around the globe. Their lives were and are closely interwoven with nature and all its creatures great and small. Our modern life tends to separate us from these treasures of the heart and soul. When an animal comes into my dreams, or shows up in my waking life, I get my book on animal medicine by Jamie Sams and David Carson, *Medicine Cards*. Reading about that animal is always just what I need to know. Resisting, pushing, and pulling just causes more struggling. Animals play a big part in teaching us humans about life and the Inner River of Peace seeded in all of us. There is quiet strength here that warms the heart and embraces the soul.

Silence is the element in which great things fashion themselves.
Thomas Carlyle

Breath is a silent conduit for the Spirit that flows through all of us. We can all meet on the waves of our synchronized breath. I have taught this for years through my Touch With Oils® Hand Massage. Silence and breath cadence are two of the Ten Principles of the philosophy in creating harmony and a sense of well-being. They reveal the Inner River of Peace that flows within. Words can often limit and dilute the glimpse of the Infinite.

Our breath brings some resolution to struggle. It turns, pushing and pulling into the natural ebb and flow of the tides. The vaporous aromas of essential oils can assist this process with The Messages. It is a language of breath and spirit, not words. Our heart knows all about this. The mind will follow. Our cells are bathed in the transformation.

Ask a specific question for a dream to show you something you want to understand. It might not come in tonight, and it might come in some way uniquely yours. Just wait and see what dreams itself into you. The act of writing it down creates a sacred synergy between your head, heart and hands. This slowing down tends to bring in more insights.

Insight for the dreaming and waking life: turn around and face the struggling situation, and breathe consciously.

Stop, Look, and Listen. (SLL) Step aside and see what is going on. What is this really about? See what insight and wisdom appears. Do you need to make a change, or do you need to alter your thoughts and feelings and see this through? Do you need to anchor deeper in *your* Inner River of Peace and wait on divine timing? Any of these decisions can be correct actions providing some relief.

> *Don't resist, pull, push, or struggle*
> *in the web of this life you're in.*
> *Everyone is in the web of life.*
> *Be there with it, in all its turmoil, and peace will prevail.*

A big part of the wisdom here is to acknowledge we don't want to stay stuck. We want to ease on out of stuckness. Slow down and simplify what you can. Life has a rhythm all of its own. The Inner River of Peace stays with us through the rapids into the calmness of the waters of our mind.

Aside from the insights from our own dreams, all wise teachings tell us to lay down our burdens, ease up, and travel lightly. There is joy and a sense of freedom here. Our load and our step lighten up. Whether we are shifting our thoughts or the physical situation or both, there is relief and insight. Call on the love in your heart and the power that is waiting. With them, comes the Inner River of Peace that flows through all things great and small.

I am reminded of:

Come unto me to a quiet place and get some rest.
Mark 6:31

Quiet times and restful places in nature are genuine sanctuaries for restoration and rejuvenation for us humans. Look what it does for the animals. When these places are not physically readily available, we must find them deep within us. Your inner sanctum is a place for this. Our imagination is a life preserver and serves us well. With imagination comes inspiration. From here, we can invent a new *holy habit* that brings us joy.

Message Six

Interpretation

What do the words "*resist, pull, push, or struggle*" create in you?

How do they make you feel, and which words do you relate to the most?

"Resist: to exert force in oppose; to exert oneself so as to counteract or defeat." *Webster's New World Dictionary.*

"Struggle: to make strenuous or violent efforts in the face of difficulties or opposition struggling with the problem; to proceed with difficulty or with great effort." *Webster's New World Dictionary.*

On family vacations at the beaches in Delaware, Dad always taught us three kids not to fight, resist, or struggle if we get caught in a whirlpool or riptide. He said, "Stop fighting against it, go with the current as you swim out and around it." Life throws us some whirlpools and riptides to be mastered.

Have you noticed that we don't get very far when we resist, pull, push, or struggle? The longer we keep it up, the worse it gets. What we keep in our mind, gets stronger. If we do force it through, it is usually something we have to go back and address again. Resolution is not there yet.

Don't Resist the Web of Life

It is a waste of our precious life force energy to spend time in the frustrated and maddening state of *resist, pull, push, or struggle.* Life is life. We can't avoid these times. We can call in the power of The Messenger and The Message to send us some life preservers. Afterall, wouldn't you rather spend time with *your* Inner River of Peace?

What does *"the web of this life"* represent to you?

"Web: an intricate pattern or structure suggestive of something woven; a network of silken thread spun especially by the larvae of various insects (such as a tent caterpillar) and usually serving as a nest or shelter." *Webster's New World Dictionary.*

Our life is certainly an intricate pattern or structure. The path of our life is a woven tapestry. The image of a spider's web shows us the ins and outs, the struggles and the flows. The idea of life being a network of silken thread, serving as a nest or shelter, gives us another image to ponder.

Look how complicated and entangled the world wide web of technology has become. It's moving so fast that even the best of the best can barely keep up with the changes, updates, and downloads. To simplify, we can choose how to function in it the best we can, being true to who we are. There is struggle and flow in all these intricacies in the web of life. Anchor deep again, make decisions, take actions, and carry on. Remember to skip or hum a little now and then.

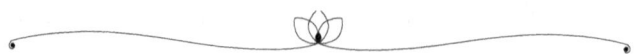

Ideas and Actions

This Message is a bit different than the others. It starts with words of what not to do. *Don't resist.*

Then it states this is part of life's natural rhythms of turmoil and peace. Turmoil is to be recognized and resolved as best we can. The solution is unique to each of us. The other nine Messages assist us with wisdom, love, and insights on how to do this. The magnificent power out there and within us is much greater than we can ever imagine. It is ready to come in and guide us when we ask and embrace it.

When we get stuck in the web of life and find we are busy resisting, pushing, pulling, and struggling, let's *Show Up and Hold the Vision* for new thoughts and perspective in resolving it. Let's *Focus on the Light and Love* of possibilities. Let's *Look at the Sky* and know there are no limits. Let us *Anchor deep* in the strength within us. Let us return to our Inner River of Peace and create the kind of person we want to be, while honoring the amazing person we truly are.

I am *Focusing on the Light and Love* for you to find your way to ease up on resistance and struggle. They come in to serve a purpose. Let's get the wisdom and love as soon as we can and move on. I'm reminded of the country western song: *I'm going slow, just as fast as I can.* I love this. It has become one of my new favorite themes in life. Before, I was always going as fast as I could. That was not the answer for me, so I gathered some new wisdom along with some new *holy habits.*

Continue to explore the best way to record The Message and keep it close. Have it in the line of sight or field of your imagination. The web of technology offers many options, as does writing through your head, heart, and hand. By the end of this book, you will have discovered many ways The Messages work for you.

> *Don't resist, pull, push, or struggle*
> *in the web of this life you're in.*
> *Everyone is in the web of life.*
> *Be there with it, in all its turmoil, and peace shall prevail.*

Your toolbox is growing with your *holy habits* and Messages. They continue to serve you in becoming more of the magnificent being you are. If this were not true, I would not be writing this book.

Message Six

Ask to be shown your way, and don't let go of The Messenger. This infinite power behind The Message does not leave us. Our call is to walk the path of love and stand in Trust. There are plenty of opportunities in life to release the resisting, pulling, pushing, or struggling. Sometimes, it seems like a daily challenge. Search for golden nuggets with all their richness along the way. Share it with loved ones who could use some gold, too. Wisdom and love appear at just the right time when they are needed most.

Honor the value of being *Slow, Still, and Simple (SSS)* in your thinking heart and feeling mind.

Read through the chapter, *The Power of the 5 Senses Plus 2*. Select a sensory stimulus to accompany The Message. Use your curiosity to find out which senses are more powerful to you. My mother wrote in my baby journal that I had a strong sense of smell. No wonder essential oils became my field of dreams. *Stop, Look, and Listen (SLL)* to what takes you to *your* Inner River of Peace.

> *Example:* Claim *your* Inner River of Peace with this Message while singing anything that makes you smile and lighten your load. Make up your own song and sing away.
>
> *Essential oil example*: Geranium (*Pelargonium roseum*) or lavender (*Lavandula augustifolia*) are some of the best essential oils for

soothing our nerves and relieving our fatigue. They also have a way to show us how to follow our dreams. Their aromas smooth out the rough edges of life and calm the scattered mind. Be sure you love the aroma you choose. Slow your breathing and be still in the gap between the inhale and exhale. Take 3-5 deep simple breaths from the bottle while thinking and feeling The Message into your being. Do this as often as you like. It is an enjoyable and rewarding treat in the midst of the worldly ways.

Message Six

Contemplative Moments

Three Steps of Vision-Making

Engage your heart-mind muscle while sensing with your vision.

1. **Set** your purpose-prayer with The Message. Ask to be shown the wisdom in the struggle and how to release it by bringing harmony into the situation.
2. **Show up** with it every chance you get with your heart-mind muscle combined with a sensory action. See the chapter, *The Power of the 5 Senses Plus 2*.
3. **Release** your resisting mind so you can recognize the bigger picture in front of you. Soften and open your clenched hands to receive the relief and resolution.

My Three-Step Prayer

Repeat anytime to enhance The Message.

1. Dear God, increase my awareness to receive your **Guidance**.
2. Then give me the **Courage** to follow it when I get it.
3. May I do it with the **Faith** that moves mountains - knowing the peace of the breath of God.

Simple Focused-Breathing Technique

Do this often, anywhere.

1. **Breathe in** through your nose, while saying**, I am observing my resisting, pushing, pulling, and struggling.**

    Pause and be Still.

2. **Breathe out** through your mouth, while saying, **I am releasing it all with wisdom and love. I anchor deep in my Inner River of Peace.**

    Pause and be still again.

3. Do three sets of this breath with or without an essential oil. Each round takes about 12 seconds.

    Can you spare thirty-six seconds right now to breathe with focus?

Life itself resembles a river. It flows smoothly, roars with rapids, gets stuck in eddies, and hits course corrections in the dams. This adventuresome challenging river trip can be managed and actually enjoyed when we are connected to our Inner River of Peace.

Don't try to steer the river.
Deepak Chopra, MD

As we take life one day at a time developing who we are, our future self is created. As we do, so shall we be. The next best step to take on our path will become clear. There is always a treasure along the way, if we believe in the possibility. Trust the ultimate source of the creation of all things great and small.

Instead of being out of sorts by pushing and pulling, may you discover the wisdom within The Message and rejoice in the freedom it allows. Life is an adventure of epic proportions to be lived to the fullest. Look up at the sky and carry on. Go for a walk every chance you get. Notice what is going on.

Postscript: during the writing of this message about my dreams of struggle and resolution, there was a full moon night. I asked to be shown what I needed to know now. I awakened in the morning (after a good night's sleep) from a dream of struggle that ended with the peace of resolution. I was able to let go of the fear in this dream. My legs were strong, and they could run. All kinds of loving help showed up to release the pushing and pulling just in time. I awakened relieved.

We are always given experiences to encourage us to anchor deep in our Inner River of Peace.

Resolution happens with divine timing.

Compassion takes us to our knees.

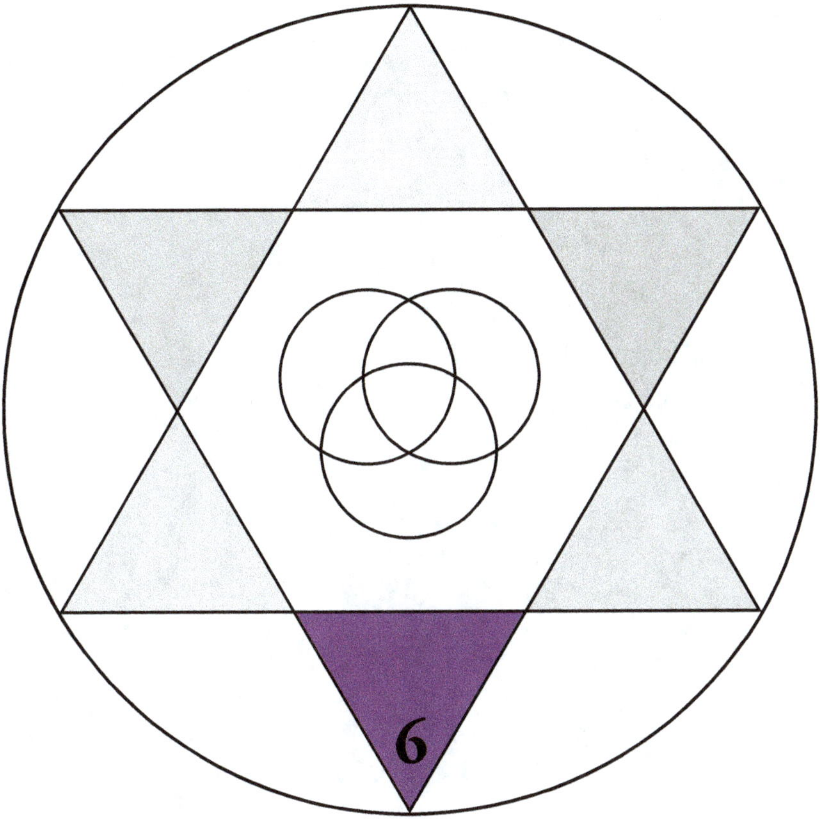

Don't Resist the Web of Life

Message Six:

*Don't resist, pull, push, or struggle
in the web of this life you're in.
Everyone is in the web of life.
Be there with it, in all its turmoil, and peace shall prevail.*

Review
MESSAGES 4-6

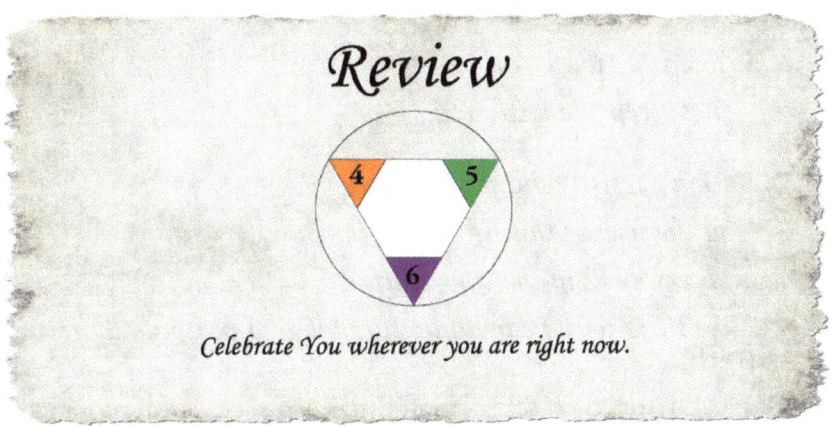

It's time to *Stop, Look, and Listen (SLL)* again.

How are you doing with the *SLL* theme throughout the book? A lot is going on when we appear to be doing nothing. How are you doing so far with the first six Messages? Maybe some new *holy habits* are sustaining you well. Do you want to tweak some, or try some new ones? Notice how long you live with each Message and which ones really speak to you the most right now.

Slow down and anchor with each Message. Be still and rest awhile. Show up, focus, and reflect on The Messenger's wisdom. Use the Simple Focused-Breathing Technique described at the end of each

Message. With ease take one to three breaths with each Message below.

Anchor way down deep
in the bottom of the ocean,
and ride the waves.
Everything is OK.

Keep Me with You,
just Keep Me with You.

Don't resist, pull, push, or struggle
in the web of this life you're in.
Everyone is in the web of life.
Be there with it, in all its turmoil, and peace shall prevail.

Used together this set of three Messages creates a sacred synergy in building a foundation of wisdom, love, and trust. Synergy is when the individual components (Messages) are used together and create far vaster results than each one offers alone. This synergy here is sacred because we are talking about our heart and soul, and the reverence for life. The reward is the growing-stronger relationship with *your* Inner River of Peace.

As we Anchor deep in our Inner River of Peace, all we have to do is keep The Messenger with us. By claiming this wisdom and power we can release our struggle in the web of our life. We merge with our Inner River of Peace.

Consider spending a week with all three of these Messages together. Know you are building strength in your heart-mind muscle.

Your cell membranes will be receiving biochemical messengers relaying all kinds of wisdom and love too.

Remember to keep this simple in a world of complexity and noise. Love, honor, and support who you really are. *Your* Inner River of Peace is always waiting to give you its best as it gives you a rest, and reveals the path in front of you—one decision-action at a time. Our Inner River of Peace and The Messenger are our anchors. Their sacred synergy gracefully sustains us.

THE ANCHOR

Weary from being tossed upon the waves of this storm,
battered by the wind,
lost in the fog,
I long to anchor way down deep in the sacred silence of Your grace.
I yearn to merge with the vast stillness of Your peace.

Losing sight in the dark night,
Searching for Your light,
My heart aches for Your love.
My mind desperately seeks Your presence.

Then comes the embrace with the spirit of Your grace,
Reminding me You are my anchor,
Remembering You never left me,
I merge with Your wave of peace that in stillness sustains me.

Candace Jean Newman

Review

I wrote this poem in the midst of a cluster of challenges. There are times when too many things come in at once and can make us feel there is no way out. When we get quiet and still on our knees and hold on, we connect back to the power of another kind that is greater than all of us. I smile when I think "Who leaves Whom here?" The desperate isolation of searching comes around to the peaceful union of remembering. Here, we find a renewed Reverence for Life in all things, great and small.

One of my favorite things: There are certain fogs that are gentle, mysterious, and almost magical. I love to see them or be in them. The shorelines and the mountain tops are exquisite places for this. Being quiet and still in the fog and waiting for it to lift always reminds me of the presence of God that is there somewhere, beyond what we can see or imagine. The omnipotent light and love of God's Presence prevails.

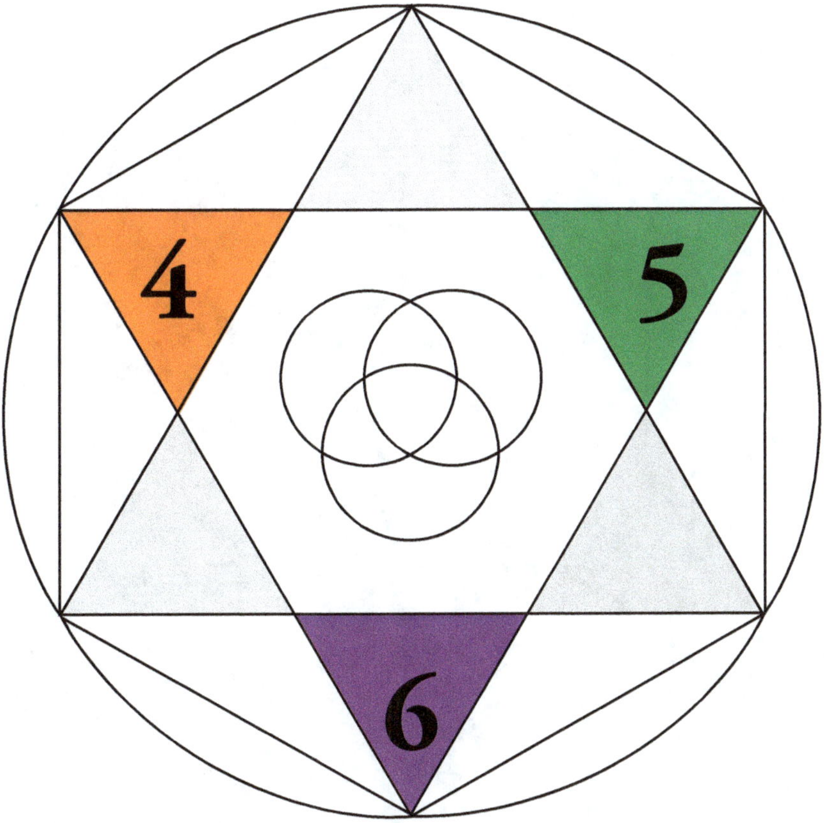

Review

MESSAGE SEVEN
The Power Out Here

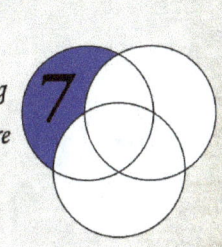

The Message

The Power out here is much greater than anything you can ever imagine, even when you Think you are in your most expanded state.
It goes way beyond that.

In other words, there is no limit to the help available. At times we get only a glimpse of this all-sufficient, ever-renewing supply of light and strength. However, by getting a flash or glimpse of it, we know it's there. We pause and wonder. The infinite possibilities have no end. We're not wired to be able to grasp the concept of infinity. Everything we know in our physical reality has a beginning and an end.

The idea of a higher power being greater than anything our imagination can fathom is a fantastic thing. The whole universe is showing up to create our dreams and more. This inspires us to keep our dreams alive. The timing is just not always what we think it should be. Remember, there is no end to the multi-universes. They go beyond what our instruments can measure, or our minds can conceive. There is also no end to the miracles of what we can do and be. Often, we hear someone say something happened that was beyond their wildest dreams.

My Personal Story

This Message came in the first time, when I was sure I was questioning the sanity of everything. My mother called one evening and said her stomach has been hurting all day, she couldn't eat, and it was getting much worse. I picked up her and Dad and off we went to the emergency room in Naples, Florida. She was in horrible pain, and I knew something was really wrong. They admitted her and ran tests with no conclusive results. They tried several medicines, and nothing was relieving her pain. Dad's Alzheimer's was progressing, and he sat in the hospital room chair thinking Mom was dying. Sudden changes like this make the disorientation worse.

I lived alone at this time, and Mom and Dad were in a condo. There was no leaving Dad alone, and I had a lecture to give at

Barnes & Noble the next morning on *The World of Aromatherapy*, an anthology of which I was a contributing author. I told the hospital nurse about the situation. She agreed that Dad could sit in the chair in Mom's room the next morning, and she would check on him. She was the first angel to appear.

There were only a few fleeting minutes of sleep that night for Dad and me, in between efforts to settle him down. The next morning Dad and I returned to the hospital, and we got him settled down with Mom and the nurse. I dashed off and gave the lecture. The funny thing is several people came up after the talk and told me I looked great, and they could see how I loved my work. Reality is anyone's perspective, only true to each through their lenses. I smiled and thanked God for carrying me.

After more tests that day for Mom, the doctor said they were probably looking at exploratory surgery in the next day or two. I was really concerned. Exploratory surgery in her abdomen didn't sound good. Her food and liquid were all intravenously administered, and she was getting weaker by the day. Trying to keep Dad calm in the room was not helping Mom.

The time to call for help had arrived. I phoned my wonderful brother and sister in Washington and Texas, and they arrived the next day. They were showing up and holding the vision. The night before they arrived, Dad and I were back in the condo, and he was more disoriented than ever. Trying to explain the circumstances to my father was not an option because it only made him more confused and agitated.

It was close to dusk, and I walked outside the condo door to stand by the trees and the little lake. The surroundings were comforting, and I looked up at the sky in a prayerful state desperately seeking solace.

Little sidetrack: The time of day was not planned; however, dusk happens to be one of the best times for getting Messages and wisdom. The energy of daylight transitions into the restorative quiet of nighttime. Years earlier, my tai chi teacher mentioned dusk and dawn are times when the veil is the thinnest. No wonder people gather at these two times a day in nature's most glorious settings. The knowledge of this is intuitive and we feel drawn to be there. We're wired for this. The contemplative spirit is palpable. These are optimal times to ponder The Messages.

While quietly standing there alone and looking up at the sky, in came The Message with its companion, the gentle wave of peace:

> *The Power out here is much greater than anything you can ever imagine, even when you Think you are in your most expanded state.*
> *It goes way beyond that.*

The Power Out Here

I looked up into the sky, trying to imagine this vast quantum field of power, wisdom, and ultimately love. There was a calmness that took over my mind. With all the overwhelm, I had lost my anchor. Sinking into a bit of despair was inevitable. The Message brought in the support and inspiration from the divine source of everything. The assurance that this power was available and bottomless, felt like a sweet drink of water from an oasis.

There was a serenity in The Message that sustained me though the events of the next week. My brother and sister were a Godsend. The exploratory surgery found scar tissue that closed off Mom's intestines. There were plenty of concerns with the realization of the rapidly advancing situation of Dad's Alzheimer's and Mom's health. Lots of prayers, tears, and miracles. There was a sense that the power and grace of God was at work here. The Message was showing us its strength.

Being together as a family and focusing our prayers on the power of God brought in more amazing moments. To name a few:

1. The night before surgery, the four of us were in the condo and formed a family circle with some drums. This was a first for my family. Visually, we placed Mom in the center of our family prayer circle with love and strength for a successful surgery the next day. Dad picked up a small drum and started tapping along with us in the

gentle slow rhythm. Suddenly, his agitation stopped. He got very quiet and continued tapping the drum. When we finished our prayers, Dad looked at me, and said we needed to do this for all the families. This taught me a lot about overloaded nerve circuits, disconnects, and anxiety. After the drumming stopped, he was back into the state of agitation.

2. Mom was rolled into surgery with one of our lavender pillows on her belly. The surgical nurse said it looked like one of The Oil Lady's pillows. Mom made these pillows for my shop, and she said her daughter was The Oil Lady®. Stephanie was one of my students. Another Angel on site.

3. After the surgery, we four surrounded Mom in the bed. She wasn't awake yet, and we used our hands to do some healing work. The doctor came in the next morning and couldn't believe Mom looked so miraculously alert after the anesthesia and surgery. Amen.

After The Message came in, I knew the only way to carry on was to focus on each happening, one by one. I was hesitant to make a drum circle with my family. After all, I had just been the Executive Vice-President of John R Wood Realtors. The morning before my brother and sister arrived, in came the voice and said I must pull out all the things I knew for my family. If my mother didn't survive the surgery, I would never forgive myself. These instructions or calls in life are things we know we must do. Look at the amazing experience we all shared. It was beautiful. With thanks to the power greater than me, I showed up, held the vision, and became the vessel.

Doing the next thing that each hour requires is the way in and through big challenges in life. It's difficult to have any clarity when we are in the middle of the fire. It asks for in-the-moment consciousness and courage to do it. Trusting in the power to guide me was paramount for any kind of peace of mind. When we show up with trust, God inspires us with guidance, courage, and faith to know when to be still and when to take action.

Oswald Chambers, author of *My Utmost for His Highest*, talks about *the Initiative against despair*. Despair is an ordinary human experience that shows up at times during our lives. When we are in despair, we don't seem to be able to lift ourselves out of it. If we are inspired by the higher power, we can anchor our trust in it and sense the absolute. This provides the impetus to:

> *Arise and do the next thing.*
> Matthew 26:46

We live in a world of duality. Thus, we need a strong anchor. Not trusting it is not an option, even when our knees are shaking and our heart is pounding. The Message and The Messenger displayed the quiet stillness of true power, and the silent strength of true gentle.

> *In gentleness there is great strength.*
> *Power most of the time can be a very quiet thing.*
> Sun Bear

As you can imagine, this Message of Power is another one of The Messages that continues to serve me throughout my life. It's here for you. Realize the gentleness of the omnipotent power of gentle grace.

> *The Power out here is much greater than anything you can ever imagine, even when you Think you are in your most expanded state.*
> *It goes way beyond that.*

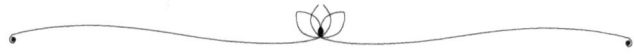

Interpretation

What does the word "*Power*" represent to you?

There are many kinds and levels of power. They can be negative or positive as they can be destructive or creative. True power is truly inspirational, and it melts away fears and doubts. There is the sense of a protective and supportive shield.

We each have our own perspective and definition of the word *power*. Our life experiences have taught us to think and feel the way we do. Then, there are the memories that pop up. This has a tremendous influence on how we each view power.

When this Message came through to me, I thought of the kind of power Dr. David Hawkins speaks of in his book, *Power vs Force*. He explains power is a source of the significance of life. It inspires us and is complete in itself. True power requires nothing, while it ennobles and unifies. Force incites polarization and is always moving against something. It creates counterforce and requires being fed energy all the time. While force consumes, power gives forth. He states that:

"Force must always succumb to power.

Power gives life and energy—forces takes these away. Power is associated with compassion and makes us feel positively about ourselves. Force is associated with judgment and makes us feel poorly about ourselves.

Ultimately the only things we can say about a source of power is that it just 'is.' True power, then, emanates from consciousness itself; what we see is a visible manifestation of the invisible."

This kind of power of light and power of love is how I imagine the nonphysical Armor of God. The word armor tends to conjure up visions of armory, shields, or weapons. Armor is a shield of protection. So how about the ultimate Armor of God being the ultimate power of light and the genuine power of love? Let us imagine here the highest light and highest love as the highest forms of power. Stand quietly in this field of powerful energy. Imagine surrounding yourself with the peace and the scope of this glorious power.

My dreams of struggling up the river and on the raft, I described earlier, were about force trying to overcome power. I kept struggling against the natural power of the water's current. The invisible energy of the whale and the horse were about the ease of true power. It was just there.

Tai Chi and karate exemplify the dynamics of power verses force. The strongest visual memory I have of this was a television special about two martial art masters. The history and roots of martial arts consist of a highly respected lineage. This science and art taught by masters is passed down through generations. The skills require demanding discipline and relentless focus. The show was about the power of soft tai chi vs. the force of hard karate. The two men were both masters of their form.

The large, young, muscular karate master came with brute force toward the small, non-muscular, older tai chi master. Both had intense focus and strength in their demeanor with the polished form and attire of a master. The older man thrust out his palm with great force and stopped the karate man in his tracks. There was no physical contact. This was so hard to believe; they were asked to do this again. The karate master said it felt like he was coming up against an invisible brick wall of energy that he could not penetrate. They both had tremendous mental capacities. One emphasized the physical strength of force, the other emphasized the ability to manifest invisible power though mastering his life force energy to diffuse force. It takes a lifetime of devotion and focus to be a world master of chi energy.

My tai chi teacher had his black belt in karate. When he came up against a Chinese tai chi master, he later invited the master from China to come live in his home in America and teach him tai chi. He said he got tired of breaking bones and getting beaten up. He saw Master Lee was simply redirecting energy and diffusing the force of karate. The master-student bond was formed. When I met Master Lee, he was a slight soft-looking man. Authentic power can be a very quiet thing.

True power of the highest is invisible. The power of prayer is invisible, as is the power of love. When this kind of power plays out in matter and form, we get to experience the mystery and the embodiment of the Divine.

See the poem in the third Review about trusting the gentle power of the flow.

How does the word "*Imagine*" fit in here?

"Imagine is the act or power of forming a mental image of something not present to the senses or never before wholly perceived in reality." *Webster's New World Dictionary.*

This definition connects the words *power* and *imagination*. They are both sourced in the invisible realm and are both sources of creation. Imagination is highly unique to each individual. The mental images with their visions and thoughts in each person's psyche are only theirs to create. There is complete freedom in the world of our imagination.

Can you imagine the "*way beyond that*"?

One of the biggest ages of exploration in this century is the ongoing research and revelation of the power of energy medicine. Some examples are the power of mental focus, prayer, therapeutic techniques, and new technologies and tools that emit and measure the vibrations and frequency of different kinds of energy on our being. Energy goes way beyond the material world we live in.

Quantum physics is about the world of way beyond. We are getting a grasp on the idea there is no separation of all physical and nonphysical elements. We are all an intricate, unique, and brilliant part of this quantum web of all existence. The field is endless and goes way beyond what we can imagine.

*The Power out here is much greater than anything
you can ever imagine, even when you Think you are
in your most expanded state.
It goes way beyond that.*

Way beyond that is whatever our mysterious and magical hearts and minds can conjure up.

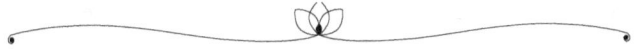

Ideas and Actions

The Messages that come to me over the years are either in my journals or on index cards. They have months and years, and sometimes a significant event written by them. They are relative to life itself. Writing about these Ten Messages has been a life review.

I am *Showing Up and Holding the Vision* that they may serve you throughout your life in a meaningful way. Writing is only one way to do it.

*The Power out here is much greater than anything
you can ever imagine, even when you Think you are
in your most expanded state.
It goes way beyond that.*

Message Seven

How do you experience this power? Truly authentic power brings a calmness of mind. There is a deep serenity. Our soul recognizes authenticity. We feel at home.

Activate your imaginal cells with all the goodness and wisdom within them. The longer length of time you live with The Message, the more you will see how many times it provides meaning. You are downloading a new operating system. Being regenerated is a thing to celebrate.

There is an endless field of powerful energy to inspire you. Call, ask, and pray it in. If you get discouraged, simply keep The Message with you and just keep responding to the call of the moment. This might be about waiting (being), or it might be about acting (doing).

The Message contains hidden treasures of immeasurable proportions of the power of love. It is always an added bonus to be *Slow, Still, and Simple (SSS)* now and then.

Read through the chapter, *The Power of the 5 Senses Plus 2*. Try a new idea to use with The Message. Notice how you think or feel. Trying something new can be revitalizing.

> *Example:* Repeat this message while you are having your quiet prayer or meditation time. Fire up your imagination thinking and feeling about the power that goes way beyond.

Essential oil example: Frankincense (*Boswellia carterii*) and/or myrrh (*Commiphora myrrha*) are some of the best essential oils for strength. They are both distilled from the tree resins. No wonder they are exquisite healers. As oils of antiquity, they have been used for protection, healing, prayer, and peace. People tend to love one more than the other. If you like them both, put a drop of each on a cotton ball. When you really like an aroma, you create happy cells. Alone or together, frankincense and myrrh slow down and deepen our breathing. Take 3-5 deep breaths from the cotton ball while doing the Simple Focused-Breathing Technique **below.**

Message Seven

Contemplative Moments

Three Steps of Vision-Making

Engage your heart-mind muscle while sensing with your vision.

1. **Set** your vision with The Message and ask to be shown its loving power.
2. **Use** The Message with one of your *holy habits* as often as you can with your heart-mind muscle. See sensory options in the chapter, *The Power of the 5 Senses Plus 2*.
3. **Imagine** receiving the power that goes way beyond us.

Three- Step Prayer

Repeat anytime to enhance The Message.

1. Dear God, increase my awareness to receive your **Guidance.**
2. Then give me the **Courage** to follow it when I get it.
3. May I do it with the **Faith** that moves mountains - trusting your true power.

Simple Focused-Breathing Technique

Enjoy often, anywhere.

The Power out here is much greater than anything you can ever imagine, even when you Think you are in your most expanded state.
It goes way beyond that.

The Power Out Here

1. **Breathe in** through your nose, while saying, **I trust the true power that is greater than me.**
   Pause and be Still.
2. **Breathe out** through your mouth, while saying, **and I imagine this powerful love and light embracing me.**
   Pause and be still again.
3. Do three sets of this breath often. Each round takes about twelve seconds. It's just thirty-six seconds here and there during the day.

Try this with one of your favorite essential oils. Put 2-3 drops of the pure oil on a cotton ball and hold it to your nose while doing the Simple Focused-Breathing Technique. This nose-brain entrainment amplifies The Message's effects.

I have often thought how the truly gentle are genuinely powerful, and the genuinely gentle are truly powerful. In this vein, I refer to Dr. David Hawkins who measured the highest level of consciousness among humans to be on the level of Jesus, Mother Theresa, and others. The term Christ Consciousness comes to mind. May you rest in the unencumbered void of possibilities with this thought.

> *What you can do or dream you can do, begin it;*
> *boldness has genius, power, and magic in it.*
> Johann von Goethe

Boldly being true to ourselves changes our life. Genius, power, and magic are words of inspiration and possibilities, and they go way beyond.

Postscript: In the process of finishing up this Message, I paused *(SLL)* and took a walk on the beach. The fog was the thickest and most beautiful I have ever seen. I couldn't see the edge of the water, or any people until they were about ten yards away from me. It was eerie, and I just kept walking. I thought how Faith is like this. You can't see your way, but you trust each step is guided. I was walking in a cloud. One time, I looked up over my head and saw a very small circle starting to open. The blue sky peeked through amidst the soft edges of the parting fog. The sky was the endless power out there that I could not completely see, yet I knew it was there, beyond the clouds. Nature will show us her power and wisdom, if we just look up and around with our heart at ease.

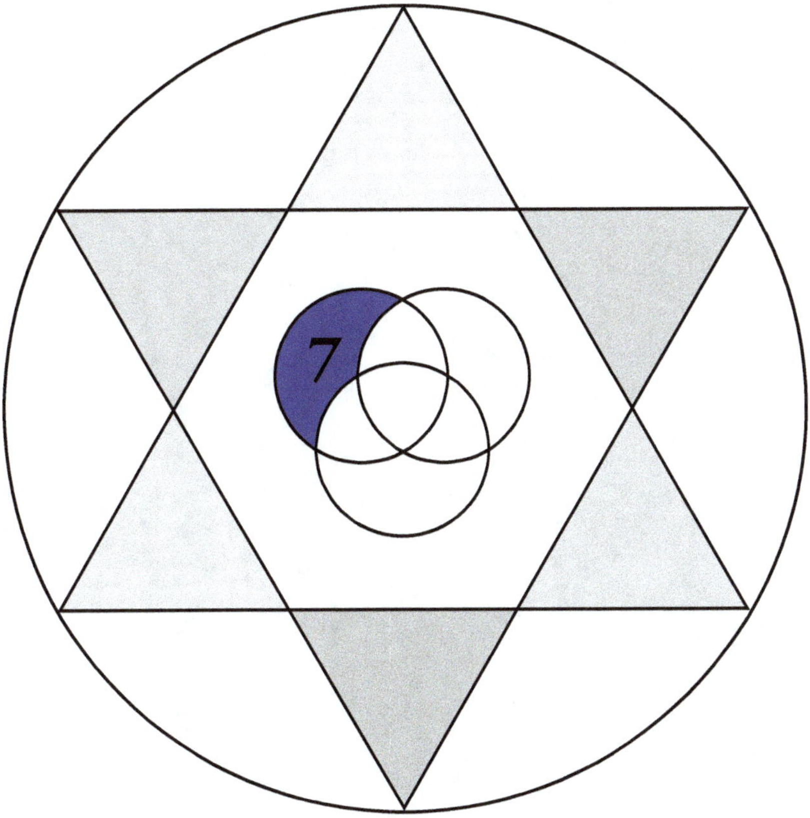

Message Seven:

The Power out here is much greater than anything you can ever imagine, even when you Think you are in your most expanded state.
It goes way beyond that.

MESSAGE EIGHT
Trust Me Like Never Before

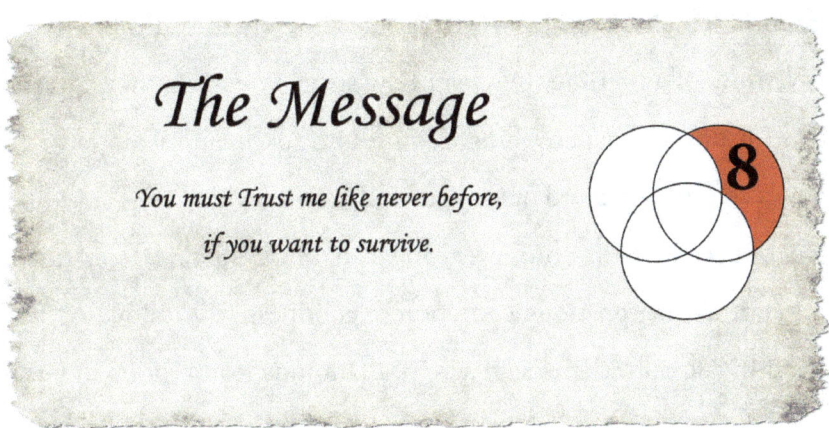

The Message
You must Trust me like never before, if you want to survive.

In other words, something bigger has happened now, and it is really time to trust the Source of the Power greater than us *like never before*. At this point, our strength on most levels has deserted us, our mind is out to lunch, and the reserve tank is empty. We've come to the end of our rope. We're standing on the edge of the cliff, looking at the sky, and wondering what's next. It appears to be the vast unknown.

Stop, Look, and Listen (SLL) with one big long slow breath. Where is your measuring stick on Trust? Do you trust anything beyond yourself? Do you trust yourself? On what level? Imagine

Message Eight

what life would be like if you really trusted yourself. The Messenger comes forth with this Message as the source of all creation. We are invited to trust the vast field of wisdom and love that is waiting to be invited in.

You are already starting to see the bigger picture and importance of the ability to trust like never before. Embrace this adventure of a lifetime. Discover how strongly you can develop this trust. It doesn't cost anything, requires no space, and is not a heavy object to schlep around or fit into an already crowded time schedule. No one can see it, but everyone can sense there is something mysterious and precious here. Surely goodness will follow. As Earl Nightingale said, there is an acre of diamonds ready for us to farm.

My Personal Story

As many of you have gathered by now, I have tended to work something until I burned out on some level. Well, I am here to say three burnouts does not mean you are out. You may be down deep, but not necessary totally out. Although, it was a great unknown at the time, as my systems were shutting down.

The situation I created and found myself in, had of course been coming on for years. My husband, John, and I moved our home and our Oil Lady Aromatherapy® company and laboratory from Naples, Florida, to Pagosa Springs, Colorado. We lived seven wonderful years there on eighteen acres in the forest and mountains at 7,500 feet elevation. This adventure was a bucket list dream to live in the Colorado mountains.

Running our essential oil company remotely with all its formulating, shipping, and teaching was an adventuresome challenge to say the least. We questioned our sanity running a mail order business in the forest, especially in winters of snow. We chopped wood and carried water. One morning it took three hours to clear the driveway. Many days, we left our truck down by the road for the UPS man's pick-ups and deliveries. However, then we had to schlep them up to our house.

After seven years of many wonderful times and explorations in the west, we decided to move back to Florida. Slipping and sliding on icy roads, dodging forest fires, and handling dry air at that elevation was getting a little tougher each year. It was beautiful, and it was challenging. We are forever grateful for this season of our life in the beautiful forested mountains and snowy winters.

It became time to get back to lower elevation and the water. Off we drove across the country with me driving one car, and John in our truck pulling our RV, with our dog Muga as his copilot. We landed in the Mt. Dora area known as Lake County, Florida.

While looking for our next home, our oil laboratory and all our home furnishings were still in our base camp in the Colorado warehouse. Maybe this would take a month or two? Well, the three of us lived in our RV for a year, kept the business going, moved the RV location several times, and searched for our home. Mind you, John and I are both the kind of people that love our quiet space and alone time. Thank goodness our love-bond was deep, and we persevered.

After finding a home, we returned to Colorado and made the huge move of stuff and the oil lab to Eustis, Florida. We had been looking for a few years for the right people to purchase Oil Lady Aromatherapy®. I wanted to do more writing and teaching. This took longer than we thought, and by the time we found the right people, we were way past our reserve, and living on fumes.

This culminated into an authentic burnout. However, this one felt more like a total collapse of my systems. At the time, we were also dealing with the declining health of John's ninety-five-year-old father, who passed away two years later. We were both spent, as life would have it.

Well, nothing was working for me. My thyroid numbers were way out of range. Thankfully, I had a very gifted Integrative

Care Doctor and a very special endocrinologist who put Humpty Dumpty back together again. As many of you may know, when your thyroid is blown off the chart, the other systems start to collapse, too. I knew this wasn't a six month or even a one-year fix. I wasn't sure if I could pull out of this one.

My relationship with God grew deeper than ever, and I committed to doing all the healing things from allopathic doctors to integrative practices I had learned and used over decades. My goal was simple: get myself restored. I wanted to feel like I still wanted to be here. I wanted to feel a spark, a sense I still had a mission to accomplish. I wanted to do this, if God's Grace wanted to support all my efforts and prayers in bringing me back.

One day after a rainstorm, I went out in our backyard and just stood there looking at the sky, as I often do. It's a big clear space and the sky-view is wide open.

As I looked to the east, there waiting for me to see it was a huge beautiful rainbow covering most of the sky. The majestic arch of vibrant colors was in all its glory. As I was standing there in awe and wonder, in came the gentle wave of peace and the voice:

> *You must Trust me like never before,*
> *if you want to survive.*

A soft stillness washed over me. This was full of hope and encouragement. It seemed like The Message was written right across the arches of radiant color. I noticed The Messenger's voice was much stronger than usual, and it kept me focused on the rainbow. Aren't rainbows God's promise to watch over us? This was important, and I knew it. This was the only way I would be regenerated, along with lots of health assistance and personal perseverance on my part. It offered the power beyond me, and I needed it. I would have to wait on its divine timing, and in the meantime keep doing all my *holy habits* for restoration. I had to let go of the fear of ill health, total exhaustion and the worry about whether I could keep going.

If I wanted to fulfill this dream-goal, I couldn't waste what precious little life force energy I still had on allowing negative thinking to feed my cells and tissue. They were already tingling and giving out. I had to move my Trust in God to another level. This requires the kind of faith Oswald Chambers refers to in his Classic Daily Devotional, *My Utmost for His Highest.* Some of the words he uses to describe devotional faith are: *rigorous confidence, heroic effort, and reckless, abandoned confidence.* These words associated with *faith* really grab our attention When one has reached the end of the trail at the edge of the crevasse, this is the kind of faith required to take the leap. The trust here believes the wings of the eagle will be there to lift us up.

With this Message, it felt like God was on a search and rescue mission and was throwing me a rainbow for a lifeline. This life preserver had a Message written on it. Whether I could follow the instructions was my assignment to take and my alignment to make. The choice was clear. Just do it and be it, with all my heart and soul.

It was time to open up and embrace the huge golden nugget of Trust on a larger scale. Not doing this was not an option. We must *Show Up and Hold the Vision* of this deep trust, sustaining us through our nurturing *holy habits*. Our Inner River of Peace banks on this. There are rapids along the way. Our call is to be curious and courageous while carrying on.

What a daily challenge this was. I kept affirming my trust. Then there would be the letting go and taking back my fears and worries. This seems to be part of the human dilemma. I kept staying the course the best I could. We all have a life that is only ours to live. Our Inner River of Peace can carry us through the rapids to the cool calm waters of grace. Then comes even more compassion for the life journeys of all creatures great and small.

It took two years to fill the empty vessel of me, one sacred drop at a time. This kind of project calls for constant self-supervision and discernment. Regeneration and maintenance are ongoing parts of life. It's also about celebrating who we really are and doing things that really sustain us. These are the things we were always meant to do and give us peace. When we do them, we feel good. However, life can distract us, and sometimes, we do things just because we can or think we should. This often means we have to manufacture the energy to get through it. I learned that just because I can do something, and maybe even do it pretty well, doesn't mean I am supposed to do it.

My heart and soul were on a major course correction for me. Everything we do makes us more of who we are. Gather the golden nuggets, the pearls, the diamonds from each part of your life, and then take the next step in creating the heroic story of your personal legend.

*You must Trust me like never before,
if you want to survive.*

The Messages in this book often feel like Mission Impossible notes to me. I smile writing this. We are handed the note in a gentle way. Your mission is declared: accept The Message with its wisdom and love. Now you choose whether you are going to accept the mission, or not. There is nothing else to talk about. Are you going to spend time with it or pass it by with a brief reading?

The good news is these Message-missions are not dangerous. They bring in a way forward with peace. Have you noticed with each event in life the call for trust keeps getting stronger and deeper? I knew my life depended on a bigger dosage of trust. There is a fine line between how much of our life events we can and cannot act upon and control. I knew I would take care of myself and get the help I needed the best that I could. I did not know what the future would hold.

Walking into the unknown requires trust like never before.

Maybe three burnouts would not mean I was out.

To me this experience was the discovery of a *Love Rainbow of Trust*. The image stays with me still today because it lifts my spirit. I remind myself to put my heart-mind muscle on walking this rainbow. Our imagination can run with this. The side effects are inspiration, new thoughts and feelings, with new words and actions. The eyes of the child, looking up with wonder and joyful expectation, create a happy heart.

The heart of the explorer piece of the "pie of me" gets uplifted when I think about unlimited possibilities. It is possible we are all writing the great epic of the rest of our life. Let's *Focus on the Light and Love* of the power of this trust. Let's see how well we can co-create our dream with its grace. This is a good way to go through the day. Remember: *Today is our favorite day* according to Pooh Bear. Nothing to lose; one more golden nugget of peace to gain. Hold hands and carry on.

Message Eight

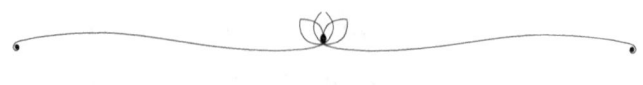

Interpretation

What does the word "*Trust*" mean to you?

Trust: From Dan Millman's book, *The Life You Were Born to Live.*

"For most of us, trust means a feeling of confidence or a sense that one will hurt us, shame us, or steal from us. Trust becomes profound faith in ourselves, in others, and in the universe — a faith stemming from a direct knowledge, not just belief, that Spirit is working in, as, and through each of us. True self-trust has to include physical, emotional, mental, and spiritual levels."

He goes on to say that when we come to a point where we trust our feelings, thoughts, and instincts, we become more aware of the Spirit working through us. From here, we can open up to a spiritual sense of love, wisdom, and integrity. However, we all know this is a continually evolving adventure with plenty of ups and downs; all the more reason to have a great relationship with our Inner River of Peace. The Great Spirit lives here.

Maybe you were told if you really want something done right, you have to do it yourself. Or maybe you don't trust yourself at all because you look at your life so far and it seems like you don't make good choices. Perhaps, you have been tremendously disappointed with someone you were sure you could trust.

What does trust mean anyway? It certainly encompasses the relationship of our self and the Higher Power. Trusting God involves trusting ourselves. We cannot put forth what we do not have within. The sacred synergy of this union serves as a deep anchor within us for life. Hang onto this anchor with your strong heart-mind muscle, all the while embracing *your* Inner River of Peace.

Trust and faith are invisible elements. However, we sense their presence, and we see them played out in matter and form. They are mysterious and beautiful. The land of dreams is made and nurtured in trust, faith, and most of all love.

Imagine what your life would be like, if you had so much faith you trusted your ability and will power to trust in the Higher Power and divine order. Instead of being on the brink of total exhaustion and frustration, you would be living on the brink of total possibility and creation.

We could move from thinking with just the mind, to knowing the endless reserve of our inner wisdom. Again, our job is to exercise our ability to *Show Up and Hold the Vision,* while believing in our ability to trust like never before. The all supplying power behind and within everything goes beyond all understanding. Exploration of this field of trust is an expedition of self-enrichment.

Message Eight

The big power station in the universe operates on different voltage and has extra big plugs. We each have an extra thick power cord that fits into this magnificent plug with ease. However, we get too busy with all the other little cords plugged into everything else. They get all tangled up and overload the circuits. There might even be a big blow-out. We know this as burnout or power outage.

Once in a while slow down, be still, and get simple with what you can. You might want to unplug some of these little cords that are draining you. Grab your biggest power cord and plug it into the almighty power source that created us. Here, we are called to live off the all-sufficient invisible grid with unlimited energy, while living in the physical grid of our visible life with limited energy. May we have a strong foothold in each world. This is a big part of life's purpose.

Learning to trust the power available to us can be observed throughout Nature. The forest burns, and green shoots sprout up again. The soil is richer than before. Flowers bloom and flourish. Mother Nature does her best to get our attention. Acknowledging and being grateful for this wisdom is another opportunity to build trust like never before.

This attracts bountiful sustenance on all levels.

What does a *"Rainbow"* remind you of?

Rainbows appear in the sky out of nowhere and without prior notice. They lift our sprits instantly as we look up and out in awe. Reminding us of our dreams, rainbows are in the sky of possibilities blessing us with brilliant color and light. They leave us with a sense of peace. The storm has passed, and light prevails.

This peaceful emotional response sends corresponding peaceful neurotransmitters to receptor sites on our cells throughout the body. The body and mind reap joyful rewards. The late Candace B. Pert, Ph.D., neuroscientist, in her book *Molecules of Emotion*, defined neurotransmitters as *"biochemical units of emotion."* Rainbows are an abundance of positive emotions.

Rainbows give us hope. They provide inspiration for our visions and dreams to be cherished within us. Our imagination runs wild here. Be a dreamer.

The dreamers are the creators and the saviors of the world. As the visible world is sustained by the invisible, so men…are nourished by the beautiful visions of their solitary dreamers.
James Allen

May we live as many moments as possible holding onto our dreams to invoke their creation. Our new thoughts, feelings, words, and actions create who we are. Let's *Focus on the Light and Love* of our dreams and reasons to be here, *and That is what You will magnify.*

Rainbows stir up visions and dreams. They are invisible in terms of being a physical form we can touch. Play with the sunlight coming through a crystal and watch the colors of the rainbow appear. Reach out to grasp it and see the colors move beautifully across your hands.

Stop - for a few moments and remember a beautiful rainbow

Look - at how this memory makes you think and feel. Where were you?

Listen - to what you can do with this memory now with this new thought. Hold on to the goodness that comes up.

Next, find a memory where you were called to deeply trust, and you did. Imagine a very special *Love Rainbow of Trust* between you and God. All of us are continually searching for ways to function well and feel good in life. Trust is a profound element affecting how we live our lives on all levels.

Each moment of our life, we either invoke or destroy our dreams.
We call upon it to become a fact, or we cancel our previous instructions.
Stuart Wilde

The Message encourages us to embrace our ability to trust the vision of the possibilities and promises of rainbows. Holding onto our dreams requires deep trust like never before. Wisdom and love are waiting again. Let's step into this abundance with our heart and soul.

What do the words *"like never before"* mean to you?

Never is a strong word. We can all remember a time saying we would never do something, and before we know it, that thing comes up and we're doing it. Then, we say we'll never say never again. There is always the next time.

This time in The Message *never,* relative to its meaning, is good. It infers we are moving ahead and being better at something (trust) than we have ever been before in life. We are choosing to do this positive thing (trust) bigger and better than before. There is an inspirational calling, a spiritual challenge to step up the ladder of trust. It is a way to anchor us deeper in our Inner River of Peace.

Do we trust our ability to do the next good thing? The way to know is to step out and try it when it appears to be right. Maybe try little things first. We strengthen our ability to trust as we embrace it with our heart. The mind will follow. The heart-mind muscle continues to build strength.

You must Trust me like never before,
if you want to survive.

Message Eight

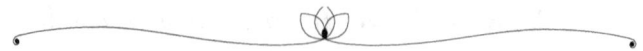

Ideas and Actions

Discover your way to record The Message somewhere, that really works with ease for you. Simple is good, and simple is powerful. Complexity and multitasking cannot live here. A simple environment doesn't serve or feed them. There is no end to how much wisdom and love The Messages have for each of us at any given time.

This message combines easily with Message Two: *Whenever you Think you are limited, Look at the sky.* As you know, the current Message came to me on a rainbow when I was looking at the sky. When I look at the sky now, I think of that Love Rainbow that asked me to trust like never before. The sky is freedom and it loves to surprise and delight us with rainbows now and then.

I am thinking about the sky, and believing this can mean something to you too, in your own special way.

*Whenever you Think you are limited,
Look at the sky.*

*You must Trust me like never before,
if you want to survive.*

The Message offers us a lifeline of wisdom and love connecting us to our Inner River of Peace. It is here for the duration and to smooth out the rough edges in life. The longer length of time The Message is used, the more you will see how it's here to comfort, protect, and serve you. There is no expiration date for its mission with us.

Build your own buffet table of Messages and your *holy habits* along with other healthy living tools you have discovered throughout life. I call this my buffet table of healing games and good medicine. It serves us well. As we change, we need different things to support and sustain us. Each season of life provides its own plate for revised choices from the buffet. The Messages with their *holy habits* provide good sustenance for all the plates.

You are discovering new ways to be yourself, as you bring this Message and the others into your life. The autonomic nervous system shifts to healthy responses due to new thoughts and emotions in your focus. A new *holy habit* is forming between your body and mind, and your spirit.

If one advances confidently in the direction of his own dreams and endeavors to live the life which he has imagined,
he will meet with a success unexpected in common hours.
Henry David Thoreau

Confidently is a word that infers having trust.

Trust in your imagination for your dreams and endeavors.

Trust in your ability to steadfastly hold on to them, sometimes against all odds.

Trust in the Source of divine timing, divine order, and divine grace to bring them into form.

As you keep this *Love Rainbow of Trust* in your mind, your heart, and in your line of sight, open up to receive the wisdom and love it offers. Ask in a quiet time of prayer or meditation to be shown the depth of this love. By doing so, you are acknowledging the tremendous possibility of God's terrain. You continue to reap abundance as you keep The Message close.

When we are *Slow, Still,* and *Simple (SSS)* we are often able to embrace the idea of a trust much deeper than what you have ever imagined.

Read through the chapter, *The Power of the 5 Senses Plus 2*. Choose one of the senses to give strength to your desire to experience The Message on a deeper level. Afterall, we are creating quiet unlimited space with new insights for our life.

> *Example:* Music and dancing are some of the most profound ways to bring new thinking and feeling into your body, mind, and spirit. They lift us up, and we experience a resurgence in our confidence.

Essential oil example: Neroli (*Citrus aurantium v. amara*) and jasmine (*Jasminum officinale*) are exceptional choices for lifting our spirits. The essential oils come from the high realm of flowering petals. Neroli and jasmine are known for their ability to lift us out of the heavy dross of life, lighten our step, soothe grief or loss, and release obsessive frustrations. Find out if you love one of these. Perhaps you have found an angelic muse. Each one is precious and intensely aromatic. Honor these dear soulful elements by using them sparingly. Remember you can always go to the balancing cleansing power of lavender, if this is better for you.

Be gentle with your precious self. Believe in the power of still and simple with 3-5 deep breaths from a bottle or from 1-2 drops on a cotton ball as your personal diffuser. Do this often to retrain your brain, open your heart, and call in your spirit.

Message Eight

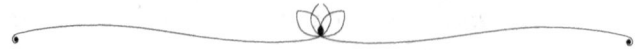

Contemplative Moments
Three Steps of Vision-Making

Engage your heart-mind muscle while sensing with your vision.

1. **Anchor** your belief in your ability to Trust in God. **Ask** to be shown this power in whatever you are doing. Let it guide you.
2. **Believe** today is your favorite day to build more trust and see it. Then let tomorrow be the same. You are building your future self. To add a sensory stimulus, see the chapter, *The Power of the 5 Senses Plus 2*.
3. **Imagine** how liberating it can feel to explore the Love Rainbow of Trust. See yourself walking on it. There are no limits on rainbows.

Three-Step Prayer

Repeat anytime to enhance The Message.

1. Dear God, increase my awareness to receive your **Guidance.**
2. Then give me the **Courage** to follow it when I get it.
3. May I do it with the **Faith** that moves mountains - and is anchored in **Trust.**

Simple Focused-Breathing Technique

Do this often, anywhere.

1. **Breathe in** through your nose, while saying, **I am Trusting like never before.**

    Pause and be Still.

2. **Breathe out** through your mouth, while saying, **I know this is the way to be guided and courageously move forward.**

    Pause and be still again.

3. Do three sets of this breath experience now. Each round takes about twelve seconds. Hold onto the next thirty-six seconds for yourself and notice the calmness.

Trusting God, the Universe, the Divine Spirit, is a lifelong ever-deepening discovery. Sometimes it is awe-inspiring. Other times we feel like we lost the connection. This is also the ebb and flow of life that we can't get around. Hold on and do the next clear thing that is right in front of you. Our Inner River of Peace flows within us and nurtures us with the soothing waters of our soul.

> *Trust yourself. Create the kind of self that you will be happy to live with all of your life. Make the most of yourself by fanning the tiny, inner sparks of possibility into flames of achievement.*
> Golda Meir

Message Eight

Pause and ask yourself what kind of Self will make you happy to live with all your life.

Look up and out for your love rainbow that arches over you and vaporizes into *your* Inner River of Peace.

Observe where your heart goes. Expect a rainbow to show up anytime anywhere. Sense how this trust-relationship grows from your heart to your mind.

You are building a castle of your dreams in the midst of the noisy construction projects in life. It's okay. We simply carry on from wherever we are. Step forward and walk along your virtual *Love Rainbow of Trust*. Try this on and hold this space for all the prosperity it has for you.

*You must Trust me like never before,
if you want to survive.*

The wisdom of how to do this is deep within you. Remember, real growth is a cycle of a few steps forward, and then a plateau or maybe even a few steps back. There are plateaus and there are bursts of joy. The hero/heroine looks up at their dream-goal and keeps taking one step or leap at a time. Our ability to trust deeply is in our human being. Our Inner River of Peace will assist, protect, and celebrate us along our way.

Trust is a cornerstone in our ability to live a harmonious life and call in the loving wisdom we need when we need it. Is there a reason not to hold onto this Message in life? Doing this takes us way beyond surviving. We shift into abundance-mentality and start to experience a world of thriving from the way beyond.

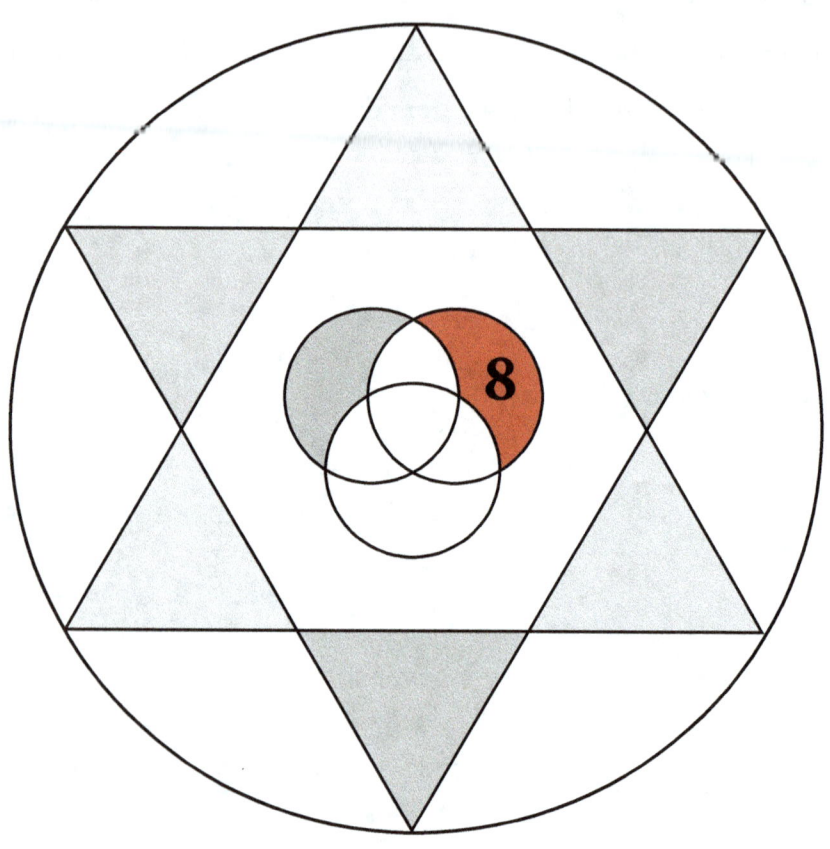

Message Eight:

*You must Trust me like never before,
if you want to survive.*

Message Nine
The Coal and The Diamond

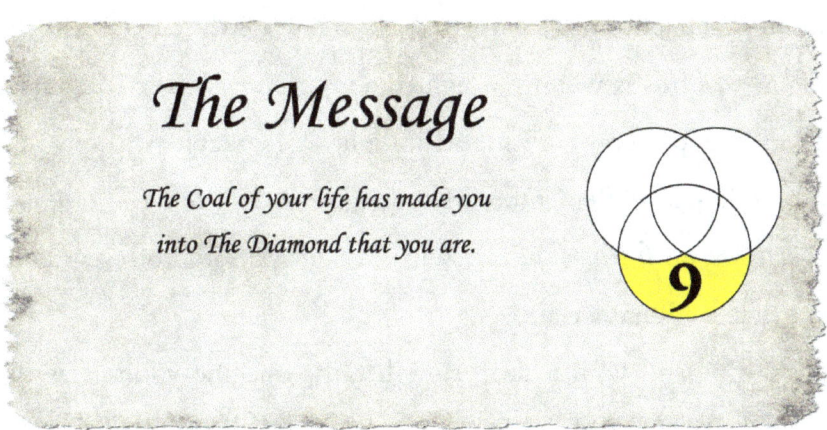

The Message

The Coal of your life has made you into The Diamond that you are.

In other words, our past with all its tribulations and tough turns has brought us to whatever point of power we are in now. Our past, with all its happenings, made us who we are today. Today makes us who we will be in the future. Our thoughts and emotions, and thus our words and actions, are all part of the amazing package of us. No one else is quite like our precious self in all our glory, living our life the best we know how.

Perhaps, it's time to claim and create a new point of power now. We are able to focus our will power on new thoughts and feelings, words and actions, and keep getting better at being a stellar diamond.

The diamond in the rough is still a diamond. So is the possible diamond that is still within the piece of coal. It is the *David* in Michelangelo's massive piece of stone. It just needs a little more buffing and polishing, with perhaps a few newly cut facets. The diamond of us is willing to light the way forward. The Messenger holds the power of omnipotent light, remarkable wisdom and astounding love. Remember Message Five: *Keep Me with You, just Keep Me with You.* The Messenger is always ready to reveal to us the diamond that we are.

Be still with a deep slow breath. Imagine yourself as the diamond of your dreams. Do you truly believe all things are possible? Why or why not? Is that really a truth? Diamonds are not created without the starting block of coal. Coal is needed with tremendous pressure and heat to turn itself over time into a radiant diamond. If the earth can do this in physical form, so can we in the many layers of our matter and form.

My Personal Story

In the process of writing this book, I questioned myself. What was I doing, what did I have to say that others didn't already know? Early one morning during my quiet time of new and improved *holy habits,* I was doing my tai chi walk and energizing exercises around my studio on my favorite moose-buffalo theme rug. Our chocolate Labrador-mix rescue doggie of thirteen years, Miss Muga, had taken her regular spot on the rug with her favorite stuffed companion, Nicholas the bear. I sat down to pray and meditate. This is part of several morning *holy habits* we love together.

The big question I was posing was*: Would this help anyone discover a deeper relationship with their Inner River of Peace? Would the reader believe it is really there and attainable for the asking? Is telling my stories have any value in assisting others navigate through life?*

The dream-goal is to show others it is possible to move into a place of thinking and feeling with their Inner River of Peace. I know in my heart The Messages are ways to show this is attainable any time for the asking and for the waiting. Life has shown me people cherish them. These universal truths are compassionate companions on our journey.

Message Nine

I was revisiting in my mind the several seasons of my life that ended with burnout, some kind of surgery, or a thyroid collapse with my nervous system going haywire. I loved the people and the work I was doing in each of my career situations. Each type of work gave me a way to share love and compassion with my clients and customers. They were like family to me and still are in my heart. Many of these relationships have become lifetime gifts.

As I was finishing this review of my past, I remembered my many dreams of fire. One particular one was a fire circle out in nature. As the fire died down, I walked up to the fire and looked down deep into the center of the black burnt logs. There was still a brilliant orange burning little ember of light. All the rest of the fire was gone. In the dream I said, *Oh, that is me! I am still alive.* I awakened drained and quite relieved with hope and belief I was coming up from the ashes. The coal was giving me the diamond of me.

Sitting quietly and still that early morning of life reviews and questions, in came The Messenger's Message on its soft wave of peace:

> *The Coal of your life has made you*
> *into The Diamond that you are.*

Bringing in its gentle stillness, it went onto tell me I must tell my story. The Message was comforting and released my doubts.

The Coal and The Diamond

There is value in whatever is happening in our life. Knowing our past contributes to our continual transformation, provides renewal and compassion for the courageous life we have led. The Messages light up the everchanging parts of our unique paths. What happens from here is each person's new story.

Slow down with this Message, and rest in the stillness of what this represents to you. The deep wisdom can be applied again and again throughout our lives, even throughout one day. Without coal, diamonds cannot be diamonds. They are formed to shine their light and exquisite beauty on the world. Diamonds are strong and stand tall in who they are. First, we must let them shine in ourselves.

At the time of writing this message, I was taking a portrait class in black charcoal. Art classes are part of my new *holy habits* that restore and sustain me. Art classes were a lifetime dream that I finally started. We need to hold our dreams closely with a vibrant heart-mind muscle until the time appears. Dreams can and do come true. They have a timing of their own. Once we experience this, there is some reassurance in the process.

Charcoal vine is used to start the sketch because it's easy to erase. Charcoal vine is made from twigs and vines as the end product of burning wood. Out of the fire of so-called destruction comes the charcoal vine of creation so we can draw charcoal portraits of faces, eyes, lights, and shadows. My portrait professor brought some to class that he had recently gathered from his burning pile of dead branches on his land. What a gift. We were creating beauty through art out of black charcoal of burnt twigs and limbs. Nature provides us with all we need.

I continue to *Hold the Vision* of doing and being the next clear thing. We are human, thus, it's a challenge. I am trusting, my next right step in the story of my future life. When I feel limited, I go *Look at the sky,* and I remind myself to keep God with me. This is a profound way to build our relationship with our Inner River of Peace. We can rest here envisioning gentle clear waters and feel the peace beyond what words can describe.

> *The Coal of your life has made you into The Diamond that you are.*

Diamonds don't appear without effort. A vision and a dream are creative starter materials. They are to be mined and cherished. It takes time. Life is precious, and you are a precious gemstone living in *your* Inner River of Peace. Honor yourself and know you are brilliant. What a blessing to have the free will to do so. Our will power is ours to discover and develop.

The Coal and The Diamond

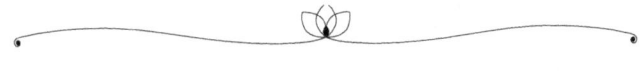

Interpretation

What do the words "*Coal, carbon,* and *fire*" bring up for you?

"Coal: ember, black solid combustible mineral used as fuel.

Carbon: a nonmetallic chemical element occurring in nature esp. as diamond and graphite and as a constituent of coal, petroleum, and limestone.

Fire: the light or heat and esp. the flame of something burning; enthusiasm, zeal; stir, enliven the imagination." All from *Webster's New World Dictionary.*

These definitions are good fuel for contemplation.

Stop, and read these again. Look, at the different ways you can interpret them in reference to The Message. Listen to the relativity we can see on different levels.

We can look at this fuel (our thoughts) as the ember of material that creates a diamond (our regenerated self) with the necessary surrounding conditions (our dreams and visions). We have an element occurring in nature (our feelings) that is a constituent of coal. This provides the opportunity to turn this hidden treasure (our new perspective) into a diamond (our genuine self).

Message Nine

Why not do this with our thoughts and emotions of past happenings? After all, we are the hidden treasure. The brilliant diamond within us is waiting to be found. It takes divine timing. It's a worthy ideal of the hero/heroine archetype piece of us on a mission to create a stronger foundation with our Inner River of Peace. The idea of seeing fire as the flame of enthusiasm (which is rooted in spirit) and zeal is an exciting way to enliven our imagination.

Slow down with these thoughts. Be still with your intuitive feelings and consider creating some simple new *holy habits* of inspiring words and creative actions. These words inspire us to expand our perceptions of our current way of being. Find the fire that really stirs your heart's desire to create the life you were born to live. Grab that ember of new thinking, and let it burn away any dross and negative connotations of past events.

You can do this by opening up and trusting the Source of the power behind The Message. The wisdom and love are available for the asking and the believing. Let this be the anchor in *your* Inner River of Peace. Ask the power to show you how to release the coal of conflicts and doubts. Move forward from here engaging and using the unlimited resources of your imagination, inspiration, and intuition. They guide you, with the love Most High, into your new way of seeing things.

The Coal and The Diamond

Remember: the dreamers are creators of the world. You are a dreamer of your world. Your energy affects the whole world. Each of us is a precious being, contributing to the ocean of existence. We are all in this together one way or another.

The big question is do you want to remain in the pile of black coal—or do you want to grasp the Diamond and metaphorically plant it in your heart and mind to be continually nurtured, buffed, and refined?

Yes, there will still be opportunities to create plenty of coal in life as long as we are here. However, now we can see it contributes to the creation of the Diamond waiting to come into form. The diamond of each of us is ours to claim and honor. As we do this, the coal will keep contributing to this alchemical process. This is a transformation and a transmutation of the grandest kind. Shed the skin of the coal and let the diamond be unveiled.

Napoleon Hill defined a goal as: *a dream with a deadline.*

With this, we can now see the word goal in a different, softer yet stronger way. The dream-goal now is to recognize and honor the past as fuel for creating the rest of our life's story. By doing so, we can live with love in our hearts for today. Finally, we can imagine and visualize our life as it moves forward. Dreams are made and materialized here. *Stop, Look, and Listen (SLL).* Where are you with a dream-goal right now? Wherever you are, just take another trustworthy step forward.

How do you feel about a "*Diamond*"? What thoughts and memories come up?

"Diamond: a hard, brilliant mineral that consists of crystalline carbon and is used as a gem." *Webster's New World Dictionary.*

In *The Crystal Bible,* Judy Hall, says:

"The diamond is a symbol of purity. The pure white light can help you to bring your life into a cohesive whole. It bonds relationships, bringing love and clarity into a partnership. Diamonds have been a symbol of wealth for thousands of years and is one of the stones of manifestation attracting abundance. Diamond is an amplifier of energy. It is one of the few stones that never needs recharging. It increases the energy of whatever it comes into contact with. Diamond clears emotional and mental pain, reduces fear, and brings new beginnings. It brings clarity of mind."

The diamond is acknowledged as the hardest known substance to humankind. How about the visualization of being as strong as a diamond in continuing to refine and create who we are, all the while solidly connected to the Source of our Inner River

The Coal and The Diamond

of Peace. This would probably be a life that goes well beyond our dreams. Oh, the places we can go.

As a side note: diamonds can be clear white, and also yellow, blue, brown, and pink. I am imagining a beautiful symphony of all of them together. This is pure brilliance, just like us.

Diamonds are like a wealthy bottomless reserve deep within us that we can mine at any time with our attention and focus. The more we keep being true to ourselves, the more we magnify this brilliance. If first to our own self we be true, then all the more we be truer with others. Diamonds remind me to strengthen my will power, so circumstances don't control me. I ask for guidance and courage in making good decisions to remind me to honor who I am and honor others.

The better diamond we become, the more qualities and facets of a diamond we can give to others. Giving and receiving become one with this kind of wisdom and love. There is soulful richness here. We are each an instrument and a vessel with our part to play in the huge orchestra and symphony of life.

*The Coal of your life has made you
into The Diamond that you are.*

Diamonds come about through transformation and they ask us to do the same. Transformation serves as a form of alchemy as the diamond is forged through pressure and heat. Representing strength on the deepest of levels, it calls us to become ferociously fearless and fiercely courageous in our ways. The light of diamonds can burn away the dross and light up our imagination. The transmutation of coal to diamonds is an inspiring metaphor to hang on to, while we get busy inventing our life.

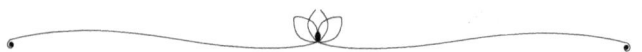

Ideas and Actions

The Message is rich with thoughts, feelings, and images. Put some vision with real focus on this for you. Use your heart-mind muscle to discover different ways to get wisdom from this. Listen to how you can use this message to acquire unique and expansive insights.

The Coal of your life has made you into The Diamond that you are.

For as long as I can remember, I have had an image of what a diamond and a rose represent to me. I believe it came about with my ponderings over a rose, and other ponderings upon the qualities a diamond teaches us. They are each beautiful in their own right.

The Coal and The Diamond

A diamond represents to me, the strength and beauty humans can obtain with self-discipline of the highest order. This involves staying strong in the heat and pressures of life. It is a pure form of self-discipline to continually contribute to being our best.

A rose represents the delicate beauty and soulful aroma that has been historically related to unconditional love. More songs, poems, verses, and art are created with the rose than any other image. Universally, it represents all levels of love. Despite the sharp thorns that hurt, the amazing flower with its soft delicate petals not only survives, it flourishes. Rose offers the scent of the heart. Of course, you must love the aroma of roses to feel that way. If so, this is a soulful essential oil for you. People that don't care for the aroma of roses often find jasmine does this for them.

The visualization of diamonds and roses have been one of my long-term affirmations: I practice the self-discipline of a diamond and the unconditional love of a rose. I didn't labor over developing this concept. It simply appeared during a quiet time one day when I was sitting in the Saint Thomas Cathedral in New York City. There was no one else in the cathedral. It was very busy and noisy outside.

As a child, when others were reading, I would sit upstairs looking out my second-floor bedroom window with a view of roses. There, I observed and dreamed as I watched over the yards and gardens behind other homes around us. Old Mr. Yohey in his big straw hat was often chasing rabbits around his rose and vegetable garden. I am sure he never knew the little girl next door up in her bedroom window was learning from him and his garden.

Life doesn't encourage us to *Stop, Look, and Listen (SLL)*. Nor does it encourage us to be *Slow, Still, and Simple (SSS)*. No one I know of has received awards for doing this, nor has anyone been considered to be extremely successful because they do this. This is an integral part of my definition of success. We must cherish and book these times in our calendar-of-doings to save precious moments for ourselves. I believe it is paramount to our sense of well-being. It reminds us of our connection to the Inner River of Peace that flows through all of us.

Over time The Message will mean different things to you, as you discover how you can apply it to wherever you are. A universal truth is a universal truth. There are no expiration dates on wisdom and love from The Messages. Our soul recognizes truth, and *your* Inner River of Peace is a source of clear calm waters. Come aside and rest here.

Coal is coal, and diamonds are diamonds. They need each other to be who they are. The process they share is a life of its own. We are not so different. This is a special exploration of new thoughts within the heart and new feelings in the mind. The

The Coal and The Diamond

result is unlocking hidden treasures of a renewed spirit and a soulful feeling of being connected.

Through practice and time, your autonomic nervous system responds with these new Messages as tools to find clarity. Feeling stuck and frustrated starts to drop away. This is the place of imagination, inspiration, and invention.

When you pause and get still for even a few moments you can be open to receive new ways to keep The Message front and center in a way that works for you. The more meaningful it is, the more you will keep it in your field of interest and influence. The company you keep, makes you who you are, and who you are continuing to create. The Messages are extraordinary companions.

Read through the chapter, *The Power of the 5 Senses Plus 2*. Combine an idea to use with The Message. There will be an infusion of their qualities. Change things around if you need to. Be curious and keep exploring, even when a step back or two interrupts your plans. The Messenger is still there.

> *Example:* Repeat this message when holding a stone, flower, laser, or another object of your choice. A quartz crystal or a rose quartz, with/or a smoky quartz or black onyx are visual representations of diamonds and coal. Read up on

them if you are curious. Maybe you want to have a piece of charcoal vine to create new beauty.

Essential oil example: Cedarwood (*Cedrus atlantica*) and helichrysum (*Helichrysum italicum or augustifolia),* are some of the best essential oils representing strength, relinquishing blocks, and creating transformation. Be sure you love the aroma of the one you choose. Use the Simple Focused-Breathing Technique described below. Do this as often as you like. It's here to serve you well. Also see the chapter, *Essential Oils as Soulful Elements.*

The Coal and The Diamond

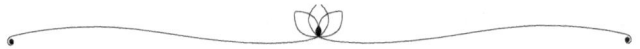

Contemplative Moments

Three Steps of Vision-Making

Engage your heart-mind muscle while sensing with your vision.

1. **Embrace** The Message and **ask** to be shown wisdom for honoring your past and today, which is creating your future self.
2. **Hold the vision** of a diamond as often as you can in your heart and mind combined with a sensory action. See the chapter, *The Power of the 5 Senses Plus 2*.
3. **Release the coal** of past happenings, and with your imagination let it evolve into a diamond of blessings and enlightenment.

Three-Step Prayer

Repeat anytime to enhance The Message.

1. Dear God, increase my awareness to receive your **Guidance.**
2. Then give me the **Courage** to follow it when I get it.
3. May I do it with the **Faith** that moves mountains - and brings forth diamonds.

Simple Focused-Breathing Technique

Do this often, anywhere.

1. **Breathe in** through your nose, while saying, **I acknowledge and honor the coal of my past.**

    Pause and be Still.

2. **Breathe out** through your mouth, while saying, **I am transforming it into the Diamond of me, one radiant facet at a time.**

   Pause and be still again.
3. Pause and experience this breathing technique three times.

   Each complete breath takes about twelve seconds. Grab any thirty-six seconds you can and enjoy this *Slow, Still, and Simple (SSS)* technique. Book it in your calendar or set a timer if you have to.

Only by searching and mining are gold and diamonds obtained,
and man can find every truth connected with his being,
if he will dig deep into the mine of his soul.
James Allen, *As a Man Thinketh*

The diamond of our soul is an everlasting treasure to be loved, honored, and supported throughout our life with all of our heart. May your searching, mining, and sowing of your diamond fields, reap an abundance of experiences with *your* Inner River of Peace. The big diamonds of peace go beyond our human imagination. How wonderful this is. There is no end to the realm of peace.

This mystery is where grace makes an appearance. Words don't work here. The soul smiles. Find The Messenger in the presence of the diamond of this relationship.

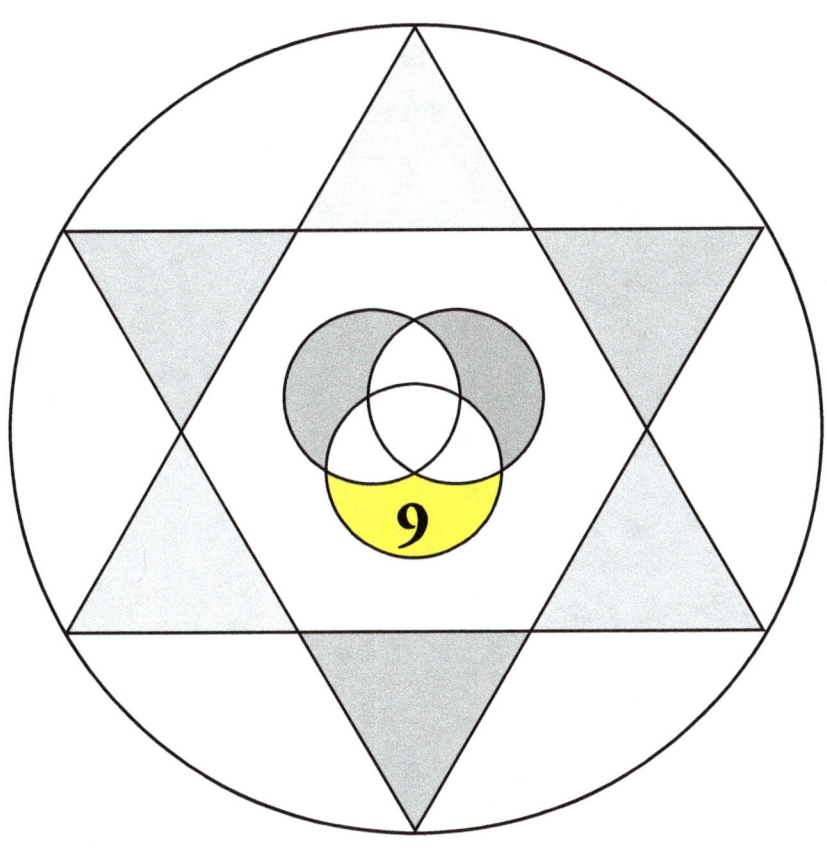

Message Nine:

The Coal of your life has made you into The Diamond that you are.

Review
MESSAGES 7-9

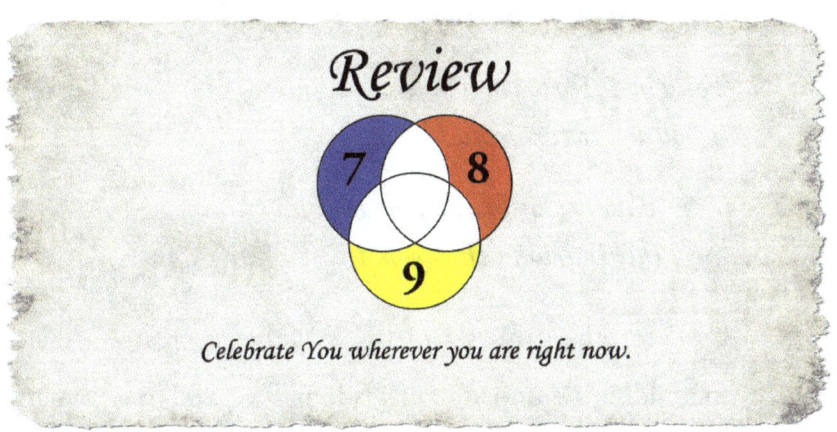

It's time to *Stop, Look, and Listen (SLL)* again. A lot is going on when we *SLL*. It can seem like we're doing nothing, or worse yet, wasting time. In these break-away moments of stepping aside of worldly happenings, we can find out what is really going on. What has happened so far for you with this third set of three Messages?

As you slow down to look at each Message, be still for one breath. Reflect on the powerful wisdom and love The Messenger has for you. Ask each Message for its wisdom. Asking, calls in the answer that is there somewhere, coming forth with divine timing. Use the Simple Focused-Breathing Technique described at the end of each Message. Use one breath for each Message below. Each breath takes about twelve seconds.

> *The Power out here is much greater than anything*
> *you can ever imagine, even when you Think you are*
> *in your most expanded state.*
> *It goes way beyond that.*
>
> *You must Trust me like never before,*
> *if you want to survive.*
>
> *The Coal of your life has made you*
> *into The Diamond that you are.*

Used together, this set of three Messages creates a sacred synergy in building a foundation of wisdom, love, and trust. Synergy is when the individual components (Messages) are used together and create far vaster results than they do alone. This synergy is *sacred synergy* because it reflects our heart and soul. It portrays a reverence for life. The reward is the growing-stronger heart-mind relationship with *your* Inner River of Peace. A synonym for sacred is *holy*.

As we open up, accept and embrace the power greater than us, all we are asked to do is trust The Messenger like never before. Claim the wisdom and love to move the memories of the past coal into new thoughts, feelings, words, and actions. It is absolutely possible to rise up from our Inner River of Peace as the Diamond

Review

of who we really are, and who we are called to become in a most magnificent way.

The Messages are treasures in creating a new operating system for the whole design of each of us. As we get a taste of what life might be like using the imagination of our mind and intuition of the heart, we acquire insightful ways we can change. Be curious and experiment with The Messages. They are only here to serve us humans. Thank goodness The Messenger is in charge.

Consider spending a week using these three Messages together. Thoughts and feelings start to change. Then comes new words and actions. Hope is back in view and more trust is building with new eyes. Your scattered parts are finding some understanding and compassion in coming back together.

Remember to keep the process simple in a fast-paced world of excess with the belief more, and more, and more is better. Love, honor, and support where you are now, and what you are creating for your future self. *Your* Inner River of Peace is always giving you its best and provides an inner sanctum for a quiet rest. The yearning heart in all of us starts to turn to joy once we experience and know the Inner River of Peace is real. When we learn to trust the power available to us, things change. There is great relief when we learn to trust the gentle power of the flow.

Review

The Path of Yearning Little Heart

The yearning heart flows like a gurgling stream
      happy and joyful to be free.
It graciously celebrates the gifts of the path.
It trusts in the gentle power of the flow.

It knows about tumbling over rocks
      and gliding into riverbanks.
It knows about the pressure of dams,
      and it has been in a stagnant eddy or two.
It trusts in the power of the flow.

It knows about cold, and it knows about hot;
the thunderous rain and the radiant sun;
the lightning of power and the rainbows of grace.
It trusts in the gentle power of the flow.

It knows about rushing, and it knows about waiting.
It knows about muddy and clear.
It gives and receives as it gurgles along.
It trusts in the gentle power of the flow.

The yearning heart flows like a gurgling stream
      happy and joyful to be free.
Graciously celebrating each precious gift on the path,
Trusting the gentle power of the flow.

Review

> God's Grace brings the guidance,
>   the wisdom,
>   the love,
>   that sets the yearning heart free.
> God's gentle power guides the flow home,
>   and shows Yearning Little Heart how to be.
>
> Candace Jean Newman

I wrote this poem while staying in The Jesuit House of Prayer in Hot Springs, North Carolina. This sweet little town had one stop light. One evening in rocking chairs on the front porch, Father George and I were wondering about the aching of the yearning heart. The next morning, I went for a walk along the Appalachian Trail behind the prayer house.

Suddenly, I felt a sense of joy, as I realized a yearning heart was to be treasured. If there is an aching in the yearning heart, then there must also be a knowing this love we yearn for exists. With this wonderful realization, on a dirt path with light streaming through the trees, I started to skip. I saw this yearning heart differently. I sat down on the rocks by a gurgling stream and wrote this poem.

Maybe the coal of the aching heart, transforms into the diamond of enlightenment within the yearning heart. I read the poem to Father George on the porch that night. What joy we shared together. Our Inner River of Peace joined us.

Review

One of my favorite things: Going for a walk (optimally in nature), when I'm thinking and pondering, is the best way to clear my head and soothe my heart. I believe this makes me a devotee of Aristotle's philosophy of *peripateo*. The Greek translation means *I go for a walk*. When we create physical space, we also create mental space. There is freedom and inspiration here.

May we give ourselves a chance to receive what is waiting to come in, or maybe it's just about standing in clear space and breathing for a few moments.

Remember it only takes thirty-six seconds to take three full breaths with the Simple Focused-Breathing Technique. Now you have created the space and time to breathe in all the goodness The Messenger has for you.

The Yearning Heart finds its home in our Inner River of Peace. From here we are able to recognize this in others.

It trusts in the gentle power of the flow.

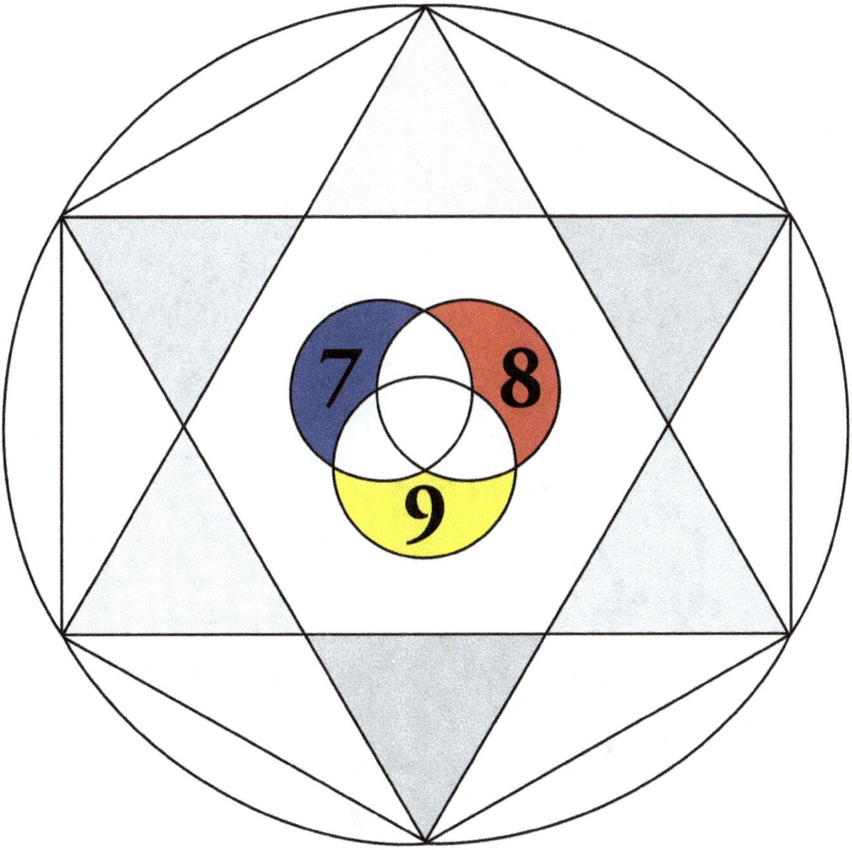

Review

MESSAGE TEN
You are Called

The Message

You are Called where you are called to experience my Love.

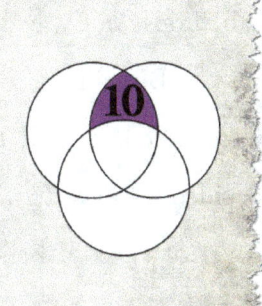

In other words, when you feel led to do something, go with the idea you are a vessel of compassion and love. Imagine the best outcome for all involved. We might not know what it's really about, and we might have some doubts about how it can work. There may be concerns about people and circumstances. However, we are called and asked to go and be a vessel of peace and integrity. Therefore, keep your anchor in *your* Inner River of Peace, and keep The Messenger with you. This is traveling lightly.

When we go where we are called, we show up because we know we are to show up. Sometimes, that is all we know. Make the decision with a big prayer to *Hold the Vision* of a peaceful and loving outcome. This sets our thoughts, feelings, words and actions in the best possible place for the vision to become reality. The energy we carry, created by our thoughts and feelings, has an effect on the whole experience. This includes the places and the people involved. We cannot change or control the choices of others. However, we can choose our way of doing and being.

Be still for one slow breath right now. In one way, you were called to read this book because you are here. You already decided to *Show Up and Hold the Vision* for tapping into *your* Inner River of Peace. I believe you have acquired a new expanded sense of love within yourself in the call for more peace in your life. My call is to provide these Messages and stories, with the vision of you experiencing the ways of The Messenger. The individuality in each of us is honored, and the Inner River of Peace is revealed.

In other words, perhaps you are called where you are called, to experience the love within you. Then you have this to give, just by showing up and being you. *You* are the gift. A new way to live your life is being rewired with the heart and mind playing together in harmony, as the heart-mind muscle.

With a sense of relief, comes a sense of ease. These new thoughts and feelings redirect our lives. The changed emotions create corresponding brain chemistry, and these new neuropeptides send their message to the cell membranes throughout your body. The cells get information about the new way to behave. Cells make up our tissue. The power of the senses adds their richness in bringing the spirit and body together. Voila! We are on our way.

My Personal Story

This message has played through many times in my life. The first time was when I responded to the call to give the eulogy described in Message Three. If I had not accepted that call, nervous as I was, I would have missed all the love and grace that was waiting for me there. I was so grateful driving home, and the voice appeared on its wave of peace:

*You are Called where you are called
to experience my Love.*

I believe the above experience was warming me up for the next event. This time, it was a *huge call* for me, because I was stepping into an unfamiliar place and an unknown situation by myself. I was going half-way around the world, and I knew I was called to go. There was no pro-con list to be made. There was curiosity wrapped in a sliver of peace with a nervous excitement

Message Ten

about the adventuresome challenge. So, I went. I look back on the love I would have missed if I had not responded to the call. It was an experience that changed my life from then forward.

My husband, John, and I met on an airplane with my mother sitting between us. Mom and I, with my sister and her two kids, were flying from Houston to Seattle to bury my father's ashes on my brother and sister-in-law's land outside Seattle. My sister and her two kids couldn't get seats near us and sat farther back in the plane. The man in the window seat next to my mother was flying from Houston to Seattle to go fishing in British Columbia with two friends. They were also sitting in the back of the plane. This was August 2001.

My mother, nervous about flying, was smelling my lavender and peppermint essential oils, and had a lavender mist in her pocket. I had just finished making two videos and was delighted to have a quiet time on the flight. She started talking to the man next to her who asked about the oils. He had never heard of aromatherapy. She proceeded to tell him about my work and my life's story. They had a lovely conversation most of the flight, while I sat quietly sipping honey water with my eyes closed most of the trip.

I remember thinking what a kind human being this was, sitting on the other side of my dear mother. John and I didn't speak the whole flight until we got up to get off the plane. He asked for my business card, and I thanked him for being so kind to my mother. I found out much later, John's mother had recently passed away, and he loved talking to my very sweet mother. They created a special bond on the airplane. I think my father, who had passed on, was somehow in on this, too.

About three weeks later in September, while working in my oil laboratory and shop, I got a phone call from John. He had just opened his wallet and found my card. This started a three-month relationship of Sunday evening phone calls. He was in a big transition in his life which included deciding whether to accept a job in Saudi Arabia. I could see he was called to go. God was literally calling John to the big physical desert at this transitional time in his life. His spirit was on the line, and his soul was calling. Little did I know I would be going a year later to Saudi Arabia. The power greater than either of us was at work on many unknown levels.

His papers to leave for Saudi were complicated, and they were delayed three times. In reading his email about the third delay, in came the wave of peace, with The Messenger's voice: *"He is not going to the desert until the two of you get together. When are you going to get The Message?"* I sat there in awe of the stillness. When I told John about this (revealing more of who I am), he flew to Naples, Florida, for three days. I wasn't even sure I could recognize him at the airport. Every time I questioned God about the sanity of this,

I was asked to trust, and then something would happen to dissolve the doubts instantaneously.

After John's return to Texas, his papers were waiting, and he left the next day for Saudi. Neither one of us felt like we were creating this, we were willing to respond to each event by showing up. We didn't know what was next. We only knew about walking through each door, one by one, as long as it was open.

We continued to speak on the phone weekly, and then came an email asking me to meet him in Cyprus in July for his first week of vacation. Sitting at my computer, reading this email, there was a pause and a stillness. I wasn't sure where Cyprus was, but I knew I had to go to find out what all this was about. If I didn't go, I wouldn't know. That was not an option.

Out of the ordinary things kept happening. Before the Cyprus trip came up in July, there was a death in John's family, and he flew home to Texas for three days. When I told my mother, I was flying to Texas for two days to see John, she said it was fine with her if I wanted to marry him. "Mom, I'm not marrying him, I'm just going for a visit!" She said, "Okay, okay, but it's still okay to marry him. I can't go but we can send your brother." This was in May and the second time we were together since the plane trip. Now it totaled five days.

You Are Called

In July, we had a week in Cyprus. We explored from the Mediterranean Sea to the ancient monastery in the mountain tops. John asked me to marry him. Now we had been together twelve days. Well, it was written on the big slate in the sky. We got our rings made there with miraculous speed by a Greek jeweler and his wife whom we found when we thought we were lost. Normally, they want two weeks to make a ring. However, Toulla and Nikitas invited us to have lunch and sit with them the next day while they made our rings. What a meaningful and fun time we all shared, while telling life stories and creating new memories.

I flew home to Naples, Florida, in a strange state of wondering how this all happened while knowing in my heart it was right. In November, John flew to Naples so we could be with Mom for our wedding, and shortly he returned to Saudi. The original plan was for me to stay in Naples with my mother and my business. He had one year left on his assignment, and we would meet in places throughout the year. Then it became clear to me that I was also called to go to Saudi and come back to Naples every three to four months. I joined him in February. My Oil Lady Aromatherapy® shop kept going thanks to my wonderful Oil Lady Elves. Mom was delighted with her new son-in-law.

You are Called where you are called
to experience my Love.

Message Ten

Usually when something is a big call, like this one was, you really have to be willing to take the whole experience one step at a time. I relate this kind of experience to stepping through doors. If you are not sure, ask to be shown the next door with clarity. Is it open or closed? If the door is open and there is a sense of peace and knowing, step through the next open door. All the while with all this door-stepping one by one, I have a Big Prayer going on: *Dear God, if this is not good for all involved, please close the next door, with lots of grace of course!*

Every time, I hesitated and questioned what I was doing, in came the Divine Source with something that whisked the doubt away. With all our differences, some part of John and I knew the power much greater than us brought us together. My Mother seemed to know this way before I did.

The door-stepping prayer is one I use often in my life. It is also what John and I used over the phone about whether he should accept the assignment-call in Saudi Arabia. It was unclear until the final door was still open. I went through the doors of the unknown again when I was scheduled to go over and live with him in February. It wasn't until the day before my scheduled flight, that the papers came through. We decided to live in the village with the Saudis, instead of in an American compound. The Iraq War started two weeks later, and we had a bag packed at the door in case we had to leave. There was war and there was peace. The year we spent there together was an experience of a lifetime. In the midst of the clashing human existence, there were rich moments of compassion and love.

This method of decision making does not mean all our decisions are great. It's simply a method for guidance, and it calls for courage and faith one step and one door at a time. It means we *Show Up and Hold the Vision* and stay *Focused on the Light and Love*. As best we can, we don't look forward and let fear and doubt creep in. It also means with each next decision we stay connected to divine guidance and get out of our own crazy way. The Messenger awaits. Thus, I have written my Three-Step Prayer for you at the end of each of the Ten Messages.

Remember Message Five:
Keep Me with You,
just Keep Me with You.

This is the walk of the heart of the explorer, the Spiritual Warrior, and the hero/heroine aspect of our life. Each time we go through a door, our faith and trust get the opportunity to grow stronger. The Inner River of Peace guides us along the river of these adventuresome expeditions in life. It carried me through the process of writing this book. We navigate one step, one door, one wave, one cloud, and one chapter at a time. We are all called in life to *Show*

Up and Hold the Vision, anchor deep in the Source, and trust God every step of the way.

We know what it's like when we disconnect and go it alone. It's a big struggle with lots of frustration. We try to make things happen, force the outcome, and deal with our thoughts of confusion, doubts, and worries. Things certainly happen that we can't change. However, we can change our stressful thoughts and emotions by holding onto The Messenger's hand and keeping The Messages with us. This is developing resilience. What are the other options?

Trust isn't easy. Trust is the way to go.

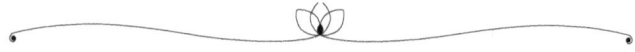

Interpretation

What do the words *"Call"* or *"a Calling"* bring up for you?

The connotations and denotations for the word **call** are endless. Take some time and think about what this word means to you. Does it bring up any good or not-so-good thoughts and feelings of memories in your life? Read through the many explanations below. The dream-goal: find a meaning that really speaks to you on

You Are Called

a deep level. This is important in order to really live with the depth of The Message.

> *You are Called where you are called*
> *to experience my Love.*

"Call (as a noun): a request or command; an invitation to become the minister of a church or to accept a professional appointment; a divine vocation or strong inner prompting to a particular course of action; the attraction or appeal of a particular activity, condition, or place; the call of the wild." *Webster's New American Dictionary.*

There is discernment involved with a call, and this is personal. If it feels like the call of the wild, we want to get a sense of whether this is The Messenger's intent. In one way it certainly could be the call to the forest, the desert, the mountains, or the water. It could be for contemplative times, life experiences, or a certain kind of mission work. It could be a real call to the wilds of the Andes of Ecuador and Peru to see if you are supposed to live there with the Inca, as I did. I just knew it was mine to go and the only way for me to find this out.

Other words that are similar to call are: *summon, request, look up, see, believe, sense, request, initiate, invite, imagine. (Merriam-Webster Thesaurus).*

Message Ten

How about this: We can believe and sense the call is an invitation requesting our presence. We can use our imagination to *Focus on the Light and Love* to see if we are to accept the call. We can *Look at the sky* and see whether the power greater than us is involved.

Life has revealed to me there are little calls and big calls, personal calls and universal calls. I believe The Messenger sent the Ten Messages in this book as universal calls. These are messages of truth, wisdom, and love for all those who are willing to drink from the well. This well of wisdom and love is bottomless. Actually, the more we drink, the more there is.

In her book, *Mutant Message Down Under*, Marlo Morgan talks about how the aborigines she traveled with in Australia would lie down with their head at the base of a eucalyptus tree. It was their belief this brought in their dreams. They talk about little dreams just for the person dreaming and big dreams for all people. Eucalyptus essential oil is a top oil for respiratory aid. It moves the rivers of the body. Perhaps with this inspiration and better breathing, eucalyptus can serve us by breathing in our visions and dreams with The Messages. It is one of the essential oils I recommend in Message Three.

A call has a sense of meaning to it. Maybe it brings in a sense of adventure, or maybe a sense of duty. It is something we feel in our heart and comes from our soul. It often requires courage, faith, and trust in our self and in God. When something is a true call, we don't have to make a pro-con list about whether to accept it or not. It's something we just know we are to do. There is a sense of a need to be loyal to the call.

Sometimes, I don't feel like I make a lot of decisions in my life. They seem to come up as a type of call, and part of me knows it is what I am to do. Sometimes they feel like an experience of exploration I seem to need, to see if something is right for me. Sometimes they feel like part of my responsibility at the time. Whichever it is, not doing it is not an option.

What does "*Love*" mean to you?

You are Called where you are called
to experience my Love.

Audible languages do not have the words to describe all the different kinds of love. There are many levels and dimensions of love. Love is something we sense physically and non-physically. We think of love as an emotion that we feel in different ways. In one sense, it is an invisible power that comes over us. If we could bottle the power of love The Messenger offers, we would have the best medicine of all.

The fruit of love is service which is compassion in action.
Mother Teresa

Message Ten

Love is a language of the heart and soul that travels on the breath of spirit. It is a silent language that speaks to us through any of our many senses. It brings with it still moments of awe and wonder.

Here is another interpretation:

Love is misunderstood to be an emotion; actually, it is a state of awareness, a way of being in the world, a way of seeing oneself and others.
Dr. David Hawkins, *Power vs Force*

Take a few moments and review times in your life when you felt love that melted you down. Perhaps, it's a sunrise or sunset, a cuddly puppy, a content baby, a special touch or hug. Maybe a feeling of unconditional love came up when you experienced or witnessed a kind gesture from another human. The experience, and even a memory of it, changes our heart-mind vibrations and stays with us for a period of time. It can become a lifetime memory to revisit anytime. We are more likely to make a sound when we experience the kind of love that melts our hearts: *awe, ahhh, uhhh, ummm, ommm.*

The love of the Most High is quiet, timeless, space-less, and encompasses our inner knowing. It is a love that permeates everything. We pause, and time stands still. We sense something is happening, full of wisdom and love from beyond and within.

You Are Called

There is a feeling we are not alone and connected to a field. The wave of peace comes in, the gentle stillness takes over, and we feel a strange calmness, we would like to hold forever. The fact that we have experienced this is something that keeps us going.

How could we ever explain or describe this? Perhaps, it is not meant to be bound by words. Maybe the mystery of existence is meant to be cherished just for what it is. It can be experienced, but not explained or grasped tightly. It is enough just as it is, and so are we. Like a liquid diamond plasma, it flows without borders. Just be there and acknowledge the grace. Breathe with the breath of God. The silence is like a holy hum.

There are times in our lives when we feel isolated and separated from this deep love that makes us feel content. We are sure we have lost it. We can ask for it, seek it, and knock on its door anytime we choose. Even when our faith and trust get tested, we can still ask, seek and knock. Divine love knows when to show up. It operates on divine timing and rides on divine grace.

As we continue to *Show Up and Hold the Vision* and *Focus on the Light and Love* we desire, then the energy keeps moving. This calls for *Trust like never before*. Then we wait, while we keep chopping wood and carrying water.

There is also so-called tough love. Maybe we are called to be shown something we are considering, and it shows us it is not ours to do. Be grateful for the experience of finding this out. Now you don't have to waste precious life force energy wondering about it.

This Message can be a very special love affair between you and The Messenger. If it speaks to you, embrace the goodness and allow yourself to be nurtured. It's another golden nugget to keep in your *holy habits*.

> *You are Called where you are called*
> *to experience my Love.*

Imagine how you can feel with this Message being part of your life. It inspires and supports us as we are called to become more of who we truly are. This is a deep expression of God's love.

> *Where there is great love, there are always miracles.*
> Willa Cather

Remember to get on the *Love Rainbow of Trust* in Message Eight. The power of great love prevails.

Ideas and Actions

As you respond to the calls in your life, do so with the sense there is another kind of love to be found. Love to be experienced and love to be shared is an admirable dream-belief. The season of life we are currently in, is the best place to explore this new way of doing and being, as the courageous heroes and heroines we are. The heart-mind muscle resonates with loving explorations.

You are Called where you are called
to experience my Love.

There is always today and again the next day to keep getting better at the joy of mindfully forming our own sacred *holy habits.* Some we keep with us for a lifetime. Others change and shift to suit each season of who we are and how our life goes. It shows us what we need when we get there. Today is today, possibly it can be our favorite day because that is all we have. It is formed and infused with the habits and routines that we hold within us.

Holy habits are powerful tools crafted with peace, compassion and love. Keep them with The Messages in your toolbox to continually serve you throughout life. I wrote this book because this is a truth for me. The longer you use The Messages, the more they become a natural part of how you are being and what you are doing—especially when you use them with the power of the senses and the soulful elements of essential oils.

Repetition creates autonomic nervous system responses to situations in life. You and your *holy habits* become one. Keep the current Message in your heart and on your mind in a way that works best for you. Share it with another person. The more Inner Rivers of Peace we can get flowing in others, the better off we all are.

Remember to ask to be shown your way. If you are unclear about whether something is a soul call or the ego's idea, ask yourself what the real reason is you would do this. Slow down, get still for a few moments. Help comes in many forms. If it is right, it will be clear at some point. Sometimes we have to wait. When it is right, there is always a sense of peace and an inner knowing. Simple and clear focus will show you the way. Be grateful for the insight ahead of time. The universe likes this.

The Message contains hidden treasures of golden nuggets uniquely waiting for you to discover them. The wisdom and love light up your way. No one else can be the diamond of you.

Read through the chapter, *The Power of the 5 Senses Plus 2*. Select one or more ideas to enrich this message. Be sure you love what you choose or try a new one that rouses your curiosity. Sometimes we just need to take a new route into ourselves.

> *Example:* Go for a walk, look around at nature when repeating The Message. Hum or sing The Message to a favorite tune. Let it be part of you.
>
> *Essential oil example*: Rose (*Rosa damascena*) and spikenard (*Nardostachys jatamansi*) are oils of reverence and antiquity. Rose is the oil of the

heart and spikenard is known for harmonizing the autonomic nervous system, notably the heart. They are both regulatory essential oils in a most wholistic way. See if you really love one or both of these. If so, use one drop of each on a cotton ball to keep with you. Hold The Message on your next aromatic breath.

Pause and take 3-5 deep slow breaths with the Simple Focused-Breathing Technique described below. The nose-brain connection is a conscious and an unconscious entrainment. This technique has a way of opening your heart and calling in your spirit. Delight your whole self often just by breathing with your essential oil. Remember, lavender is always a choice, and a drop can be added to rose or spikenard.

See ideas for more ways to use the essential oils in the chapter, *Essential Oils as Soulful Elements*.

Message Ten

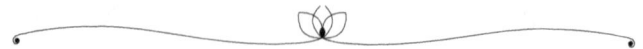

Contemplative Moments

Three Steps of Vision-Making

Engage your heart-mind muscle while sensing with your vision.

1. **Align** your heart with The Message and ask for clarity about the call.
2. **Keep** The Message connected to your heart-mind muscle combined with an essential oil sensory action. See the chapter, *The Power of the 5 Senses Plus 2*
3. Know in your heart there is **Love** to be found when we are **Called**. Believe ahead of time you are receiving the abundance. It may surprise you.

Three-Step Prayer

Repeat anytime to enhance The Message.

1. Dear God, increase my awareness to receive your **Guidance** as I step through each door.
2. Then give me the **Courage** to follow it and step through the next open door.
3. May I do it with the **Faith** that moves mountains - and knows only Love.

You Are Called

Simple Focused-Breathing Technique

Do this often, anywhere.

1. **Slowly breathe in** through your nose, while saying**, I am responding to the Call.**

    Pause and be Still.

2. **Slowly breathe out** through your mouth, while saying, **and I am experiencing Love.**

    Pause and be still again.

3. Try three sets of this twelve second breath and enjoy the next thirty-six seconds.

Life is without a doubt a challenging adventure. It's a smoother trip when we are connected to our Inner River of Peace. This is a lifelong dream-goal and full of opportunities to uncover golden nuggets and diamonds of holy happenings. When we agree to respond to the call as a vessel of compassion and love, God can show us wonderful things.

> *Compassion is by nature gentle, peaceful and soft,*
> *but is very powerful.*
> Dalai Lama

Your Inner River of Peace is a compassionate place of love, the water flows gently, and the power of this water conquers all. Travel through life with one foot firmly planted in *your* Inner River of Peace. This is the love that is within you.

*You are Called where you are called
to experience my Love.*

Be full-of-thanks and appreciation every chance you get. Life is precious—and so are you.

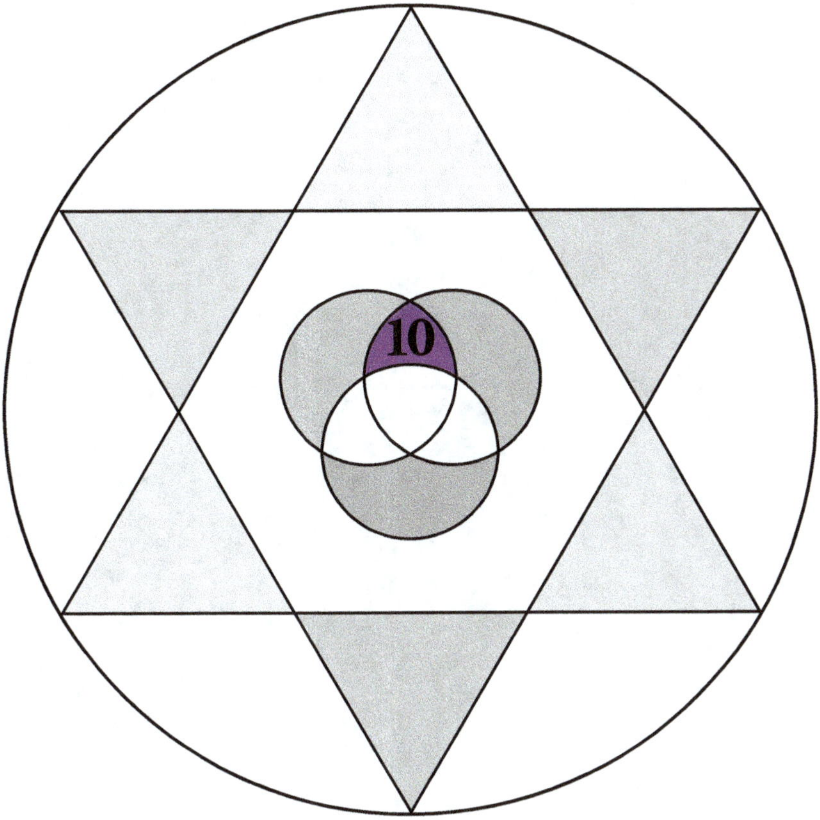

Message Ten:

*You are Called where you are called
to experience my Love.*

REVIEW
MESSAGES 1-10

Review

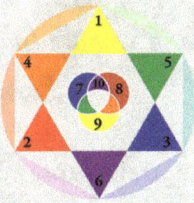

Celebrate You for all that you are right now with these Ten Messages of Love in your heart, mind, and all the rest of wonderful you.

Find some quiet time to stop and look through the book, slowly or quickly. Listen to what The Messages have to say at this point. It may be different from the first time you visited them because you are different. Are there Messages that really speak to you? Have you created some *holy habits*? Reflect on what has happened and be full of thanks. When the frustrations and confusion rear their heads, just remember to fret not.

> *What are you fretting about? Don't you remember?*
> *All YOU agreed to do is:*
> *Show Up and Hold the Vision.*
> *We can do all the rest through you.*   *Message One*

Review

Notice how the Ten Messages create a highly effective performance team. They are here to be of royal service to all of us. The sacred synergy they create together is an adventure of a lifetime. The Messenger offers us a place in our hearts to dwell, with a mission to show us the way forward. This offering of Love is simply waiting for each of us to come home to our new heart-mind place of peace, where everything we have ever dreamed of exists and is nurtured.

> *Whenever you Think you are limited,*
> *Look at the sky.*   *Message Two*

This book is an invitation to embrace The Messenger and The Messages that are here for you. Imagine you have been on an inspirational secret mission-journey that continues to reveal more of your majestic self. This brilliant magnificent Inner River of Peace is actually you. With childlike eyes of wonder, let your intuition show you ways to keep your *holy habits* with Ten Messages of Love in your life. Honor your past, compassionately live your present, and support your future with the amazingly glorious power of the Great Holy Spirit that is available.

> *Focus on the Light and Love*
> *and That is what You will magnify.*   *Message Three*

There is a time to take action and a time to take a break. Do and Be, act and rest, think and feel, all are meant to be partners-in-balance and cycles of life. This is a real challenge in a world of complexity with all its demands. The cacophony of happenings and noise bombards our nervous system and rattles our spirit. It can actually reprogram our central nervous system to thinking this state of unrest is normal.

> *Anchor way down deep*
> *in the bottom of the ocean,*
> *and ride the waves.*
> *Everything is okay.*   *Message Four*

Any tools we gather as new *holy habits*, remind us to take a deep slow breath for a few moments and be still. Then we realize there are simple things we can do to connect to our Inner River of Peace. The seat of wisdom and love, compassion, and thankfulness offer us a spot to regenerate, one breath and one hour at a time.

> *Keep Me with You,*
> *just Keep Me with You.*   *Message Five*

We live in a world of duality, so the seasons of life have their own unique rough and smooth waters. The winds of change come in, and they go out.

> *Don't resist, pull, push, or struggle*
> *in the web of this life you are in.*
> *Everyone is in the web of life.*
> *Be there with it, in all its turmoil, peace shall prevail.*
>   *Message Six*

Life will throw us times when we think the challenge is impossible to handle. Overwhelm can take over, and we can barely keep our heads above water.

> *The Power out here is much greater than anything*
> *you can ever imagine, even when you Think you are*
> *in your most expanded state.*
> *It goes way beyond that.* — *Message Seven*

Each time we feel unsure of our ability to come back from burnout, or get through a long time of drought, or simply make it through the day, we can remember the field of infinite possibilities. This field is beyond us and within us. We are part of the field, and it is a big leap of faith to surrender to it.

> *You must Trust me like never before,*
> *if you want to survive.* — *Message Eight*

In finding out more and more of who we are and being true to our whole self on all levels, we must *Stop, Look, and Listen (SLL)* to our life now and then. Step aside and observe your life so far. Then we can see some different choices for new thoughts and feelings as we go forward. The call is to honor our past experiences for making us who we are and who we can become. As we do this and live each day with a diamond in our heart, we create the story of our future.

Review

> *The Coal of your life has made you*
> *into The Diamond that you are.*   *Message Nine*

Giving and receiving become one when we come from the powerful place of love and compassion. Responding to our call each day is a worthy dream-goal of challenging and amazing adventures as we navigate the waters of life. We were formed and born in water. Somehow, we innately know how to do and be this.

> *You are Called where you are called*
> *to experience my Love.*   *Message Ten*

Bringing the ten Messages into our lives is a conscientiously conscious decision to embrace the wisdom and love The Messenger offers us.

- The geometric symbol represents the sacred synergy of these Ten Messages of Love. This serves as a power grid to bring our scattered parts back together as we anchor in our Inner River of Peace.
- It is a visual authentic color wheel of the artist's palette, offering primary, secondary and tertiary colors in different geometric shapes and sizes, honoring the seasons of our lives.
- As a Message Mandala, it guides us home into the center of our inner sanctum. Each Message has its place in the *Circle of Compassion in Action* that encompasses the symbol, loving

Review

and protecting us each step of the way. Sacred geometry flows through the Inner River of Peace.

This geometric symbol is also the grid and mandala for the Ten Principles philosophy and the Motions of Stillness of our Touch With Oils® Methods. The color wheel and mandala are indicative of the many levels and dimensions within us and in life.

Seeing something in black and white, and then seeing it in color, creates different thoughts and feelings. I present this Message Mandala to you each way. Pause here with the Simple Focused-Breathing Technique and the essential oil you love while gazing at the geometric symbol. See how many different shapes you can find. Honor any thoughts, feelings, and memories that arise.

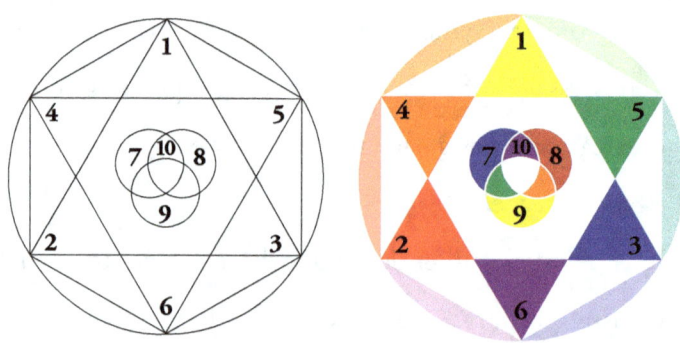

See this as part of the strength and peace that is supporting you and offering you the sense of an inner harmonious belonging. All these pathways support each other and build a strong foundation for us to build upon each day and season of our life. Together they

Review

create a unique sacred synergy to provide many loving ways to bring harmony into our lives in a world of duality.

Here we find the true meaning of holding a reverence for life in all things, which starts with holding reverence for our own life. Being still with gratitude is the giving and receiving that becomes one in the complete circle of life.

Here are some possible ways to see The Messages:

1. I am Showing Up and Holding the Vision of being a vessel of peace, compassion, and love.
2. When I Think I am limited, I Look at the sky, and see the endless field of infinite possibilities.
3. I Focus on the Light and Love, and That is what I magnify today.
4. I Anchor deep in my Inner River of Peace and ride out the waves of turmoil.
5. I Keep You with Me, I just Keep You with Me, and I know everything is okay.
6. I don't resist, pull, push or struggle. I acknowledge the web of life, and embrace new thoughts, feelings, words and actions for my Inner River of Peace.
7. I embrace the Power much greater than me and I ask to be shown the way.
8. I Trust like never before, and I walk the *Love Rainbow of Trust*.

Review

9. I honor my past as The Coal that has made me into The Diamond I am now. I cherish my future.

10. I am Called where I am called, to experience only the Love of God, the Source, the Great Holy Spirit. I show up with this vision with my heart-mind muscle, and I am grateful.

Invite The Messages into the sacred temple of your heart. Let your magical and mysteriously brilliant mind embrace them. Be true to who you really are and live from *your* Inner River of Peace. Perhaps, this is the God Particle within each of us that sustains us. The more we focus on it, the deeper the reservoir. Life is precious, and so are you.

The Purple Sea

Undulating rhythms of the wind
Riding their way through rows of Lavender
On the endless purple sea.

Rippling waves of green stems and leaves
Crested with purple flowers
Uniting the heart and soul
In a field of unbounded dreams.

The sacred hum of the bumble bees
The sounds and colors of the wind
The harmony of ebb and flow.

Review

> Here lives the gentle breeze of peace
> In a field of endless love
> A holy place to meet
> Our Inner River of Peace.
>
> Candace Jean Newman

In July of 1995, it was with the pure joy of a child to visit the Norfolk Lavender Fields in England with John Black of Aroma Trading Limited. I have always found great inspiration in quiet and in nature. Standing there amongst a hundred acres of blooming lavender, it brought to mind William Wordsworth's explanation of what creates poetry: *a spontaneous overflow of powerful emotion.* Years earlier I had visited his cottage in the Lake District of England. I wrote this poem on my way back home across the ocean from Norfolk. The Lavender Fields felt like another home.

> *When you do things from your soul,*
> *you feel a river running through you.*
>
> Rumi

May you do this book from your soul and feel *your* Inner River of Peace running through you. This is a new and improved way to be. Tap, walk, dance, sing, and smell your way into each scene and act you are writing for your role on the stage of life. Be sure to *Show Up and Hold the Vision* each day for new and improved ways of thinking, feeling, speaking and acting.

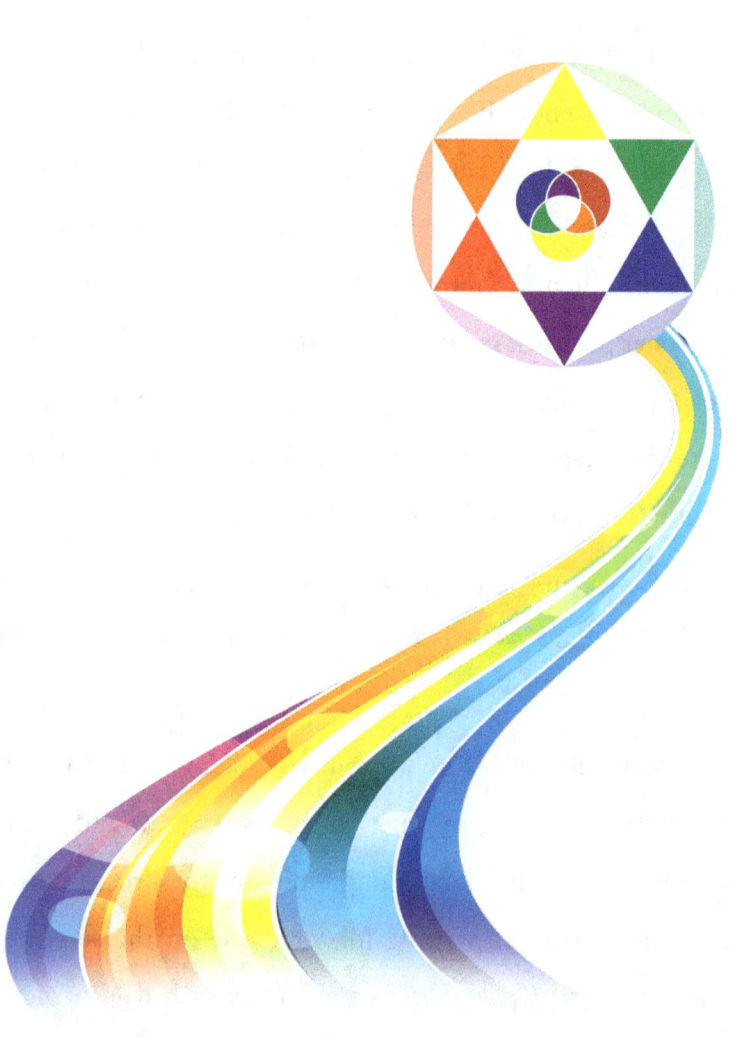

The Power of the 5 Senses Plus 2

*If we believe the body is in the soul and the soul is divine ground,
then the presence of the divine is completely here, close to us.
Being in the soul, the body makes the senses thresholds of soul.*
John O'Donahue, *Anam Cara*

Nature first taught us humans about the value of the senses. Survival and pleasure depended upon tasting berries, smelling flowers, touching water, seeing natural sights, and hearing animals and thunder. Many of our scents now are man-made. Returning to soulful natural elements is an integral part of being in *your* Inner River of Peace. Let your cells dance and be bathed by the senses and beauty of nature.

There have been volumes written for centuries about our five senses. They are sensational, fascinating, and mysterious. They have the ability to show us the beauty of life and inspire us to dream and create. As the author, I have taken the liberty of including my own twist by adding two more senses: movement and intuition/imagination. This is the results of the seven decades of my life experiences thus far.

Our senses are powerfully connected to us in many ways. The comingling of the senses helps bring our scattered parts back together, while assisting our continual healing and enlightenment on many levels. In regard to this writing, we are viewing our senses as portals to our wholeness. Thus, the intention is to experience them with integrity in a holy way. Our senses are a vehicle, *thresholds*, connecting us to our soul. When experienced in this manner, our senses act as soulful elements waiting to be asked to serve with The Messages. Together they merge in their mission to guide us home to our Inner River of Peace. This place of reverent stillness is within us. From here, we can hear what we are to know next.

These seven sensual pathways can simultaneously shift our thoughts, feelings, words, and actions. They provide an integral foundational piece in the self-realization of the precious gift each of us truly is. The unlimited field of the potentiality of our senses offers profound ways to remind us to *Stop, Look, and Listen (SLL)*. As we create some *holy habits* with deep mindfulness, our heart-mind muscle is enriched. Sometimes the call is to slow down, be still and remember the strength in simple. This is liberating and shows us the highly productive path of knowing when to wait and when to act.

This presentation is an offering of suggestions. Simply be open and receive any goodness that is here for you. There are so many beautiful ways to use our senses to further expedite and assimilate the meaning of The Messages. This assimilation allows for the wisdom and love of each Message to go deeper and quicker into our whole being on a cellular level. With these new thoughts and emotions, simultaneously creating new brain chemistry, our cells are bathed with new information. This chain of reactions has a way of its own in opening our hearts and calling in our spirit. The Presence of our Soul appears on a wave of peace.

When we feel peace, our brain puts out neuropeptides of peace as the result of this emotion. Perhaps when the cell membranes receive these new neuropeptides of peace, they say to the cells: *Hey, what are you doing? You don't have to be angry or frustrated anymore, you can shift to peaceful feelings.* This is scientifically proven as a physiological brain-to-cell response, with the new science of epigenetics. Why would we not explore this with great curiosity and wonder?

Imagine what your life would be like, if you exchanged even just one of your frustrating struggles for the freedom of fluidity? What about exchanging some limited expectations and judgments for compassion and understanding? Oh, my goodness, how wonderful *this* sounds. It's often one sacred step at a time, unless God gives us one big heart-pumping leap. Whichever it is, anchor deep in *your* Inner River of Peace and cherish the respite of smooth waters. This is an oasis in what sometimes feels like the desert of life. Be full of thanks as often as you can. This spreads delightfulness into your world, and the whole world.

There is information in each Message that personally relates to you. With a mindset of childlike wonder and curiosity, try some ideas and learn more about your wonderful Self. Nurturing your mind and body creates the side effects of a more harmonious life. Discover how using one or more of your senses, enhances each Message. Focus on simple and enjoyable ways to use your senses, to get you thinking with your heart and feeling with your mind.

New thoughts, feelings, and memories come up as you combine a Message with a sensory stimulus. We know the power of smell or a song can instantly pop up a memory, even one we may have forgotten. When an old memory pops up, good or not so good, it tells us how we are doing with that memory. Eventually, they can grow, soften, dissipate, or vaporize. Anchor deep with The Messenger and observe the waves of life events and the clouds of emotions.

Select positive sensory experiences to amplify the goodness and guidance The Messages offer. This brings us home to our true self on what Paulo Coelho calls the *Path of our Personal Legend*. Remember to contemplate with new eyes. Let The Message, with your senses, assist you.

The past is gone. Turn around and embrace what it has for you now and lift it up with as much grace as possible.

> *The Coal of your life has made you*
> *into The Diamond that you are.*   *Message Nine*

The future is not known. Imagine and visualize how you see yourself living it.

> *Whenever you Think you are limited,*
> *Look at the sky.*   *Message Two*

The present is right now. This can be the beginning of the new story you are living, hour by hour the best that you can. The next now is another chance to create, do and be from this new perspective of yourself. What ways bring you peace?

> *What are you fretting about? Don't you remember?*
> *All YOU agreed to do is:*
> *Show Up and Hold the Vision.*
> *We can do all the rest through you.*   *Message One*

Any little or big changes matter. One by one, we take our next step. In doing so, we build our path forward. Just keep heading in the right direction with the next sacred step. Ask The Messenger for insights and guidance. The Messages are life preservers bringing feelings of self-control back into your life. You are the only person in charge of your Inner River of Peace. Master your connection with this loving companion. With enough repetition, water can smooth down the rough stone-edges of life.

> *Keep Me with You,*
> *just Keep Me with You.*   Message Five

How it works

Whether we use one sense or several with The Message, they move the insights from the intellectual level into the cellular level. With this in mind, one sense can be enough. As the synergy created vibrates through the fabric of our being, it changes our thoughts and feelings. The wisdom and love keep growing deeper with repetition and time.

Our perspective widens as we age with these universal Messages of Love that do not age with time. They don't know about what we call "time." What an exciting way to live out our lives! This is often a daily or hourly adventuresome challenge. It is the way of hope, faith, and most of all the kind of love for which our hearts yearn.

Example: we can intellectually know that if we *Focus on the Light and Love (Message Two),* it will be magnified in our life. However, how do we get it on a cellular level in order to really believe it and have the body really feel it? The Messages are reinforced with sensory stimuli as they rewire our brain. It calls for our heart-mind muscle to engage and become stronger. We must *Show Up and Hold the Vision* for doing and being our part.

1. Know that you *really* want to think and feel The Message's wisdom in the fabric of your being.
2. Keep the current Message with you and see it at least 1-3 times a day.
3. Use any of the senses to fast-track it into the many levels of who you are. Let it take you home to your heart. The mind will follow. Select one sense and keep it simple or combine several if you wish. Let your spirit sparkle with Trust, like never before.

Read the options and see what you might want to try. By using these throughout my life on a mission to feel better, I realized we all want to feel better in some way. This means we are on an adventuresome expedition in search of our Inner River of Peace. We each have our own unique and beautiful inner river to explore.

In creating your own healing games and good medicine, you are developing a ritual that is meaningful and do-able in your life. There are many connotations that come up for each of us with the word *ritual*. I love Kent Nerburn's definition in his lovely little book, *Small Graces*. Let's visit this again right now:

> *Ritual is routine infused with mindfulness.*
> *It is habit made holy.*

Our cup of coffee in the morning is a routine, and when infused with mindfulness becomes a *holy habit*. It is certainly a favorite ritual of mine. Making coffee or tea can become a very meaningful experience. Add one of The Messages to this special occasion as you smell and taste the coffee or tea. Consider adding one of The Message Reviews to this holy time. Holding the cup with your hands, feel the warmth, and breathe in the aroma before you taste it. Slow down and be still. You might want to breathe with the Simple Focused-Breathing Technique described at the end of each Message. Exhale with an *Ahhh* and take a sip. Sip by sip, you're on your way with *your* Inner River of Peace intact.

The three senses of smell, touch, and taste comingle in the *holy habit* of coffee or teatime with a Message. This is fun and delicious! Try this with a *holy habit* of eating, too. Bite by bite. This means we are actually tasting the food. Yum, yummy, and yummier.

Here are a few more examples that strengthen your heart-mind muscle with the senses and The Messages:

1. Combine your Message with a form of movement in the morning, such as, walking, yoga, biking, tai chi, running, or weightlifting.
2. Breathe and/or do an isometric with The Message throughout the day. Isometrics can be done anywhere by squeezing and releasing any muscle while breathing into it. No one can see what you are doing. Hands, feet, or abdominals are my simple ones while standing in the grocery line.
3. Use The Message with sound in the morning or night. I use soft flute music with tai chi prayer walking in my studio. When I sit down, my chocolate-lab-mix doggie, Muga, brings her toy and lays quietly while I pray and meditate. What a precious prayer partner! This is a heartfelt example of a healing game and good medicine.

Choose something that lifts your spirit just to think about it. Be curious and try it. The idea is to enjoy the *holy habits* of your very own creation.

It is possible to get our minds outside the box of preconceived limits we carry within us by using the amazing, miraculous parts of our brain, heart, and spirit. In this unlimited field of possibilities, we tap into our intuitive intelligence and our imaginative wisdom.

Or, maybe it is imaginative intelligence and intuitive wisdom? It's both, and it's everything.

The wonderful news is the simultaneous brain-body response from The Message's wisdom and love, along with a sensory stimulus, happens without real effort on our part at all. Our autonomic nervous system is in favor of this way of being. Here we find the starting engine for the shift into embracing more of our miraculous self.

Our Five Senses

Our senses allow us to experience life as we know it. They are hardwired in the brain, creating instantaneous emotional reactions with corresponding brain chemistry. It happens automatically from the thoughts, feelings, and memories the senses stir up or the new ones created. Responses to the senses live in the mysterious limbic system, the seat of our emotional brain.

> *"Most people think of the mind as being located in the head, but the latest findings in physiology suggest that the mind doesn't really dwell in the brain but travels the whole body on caravans of hormone and enzyme, busily making sense of the compound wonder we catalogue as touch, taste, smell, hearing and visions. There is no way in which to understand the world without first detecting it through the radar-net of our senses."*
> Diane Ackerman, *A Natural History of the Senses*

People that are deprived of one or more senses often suffer from various types of depression. They have lost a meaningful and joyful way to relate to their world. This is especially true if they were born with the sense and then lost it. The remaining senses often become stronger.

Funk & Wagnall's New College Standard Dictionary defines *sense* as:

"The faculty of sensation; sense perception. In general, any of certain agencies by or through which an individual receives impressions of the external world; popularly one of five senses. Any receptor or group of receptors, specialized to receive or transmit stimuli, either external as of sight, sound, smell, etc., or internal, as of hunger, thirst, sex, equilibrium, muscular and visceral movements, etc."

Our five senses started with the Aristotelian division of senses into sight, sound, smell, taste, and touch. They enrich our lives, sweeten our hearts, and show us how to really survive and joyfully thrive. What beautiful companions our senses make for The Messages.

Our Sense of Smell

Smell is a potent wizard that transports us across thousands of miles and all the years we have lived.
Helen Keller

I love this *potent wizard* in essential oils. One of my favorite things to do in my aromatherapy classes is to pass around smelling sticks charged with 1-2 drops of a genuine single essential oil. I observe the students and then ask if anyone would share their nose-brain emotional responses.

The range of responses from the aroma of tea tree included sweaty horse leather, stinky socks, and too medicinal. Tea Tree tends to bring up some harsher type comments. I see a lot of squished-up faces. One time, I saw a man in the back of the room with a soft smile on his face. He looked like he just smelled the peace of lavender. I asked him where he had gone. "This reminds me of my grandfather. When I was five years old, he took me on walks through the woods on a dirt path. I can smell the forest." He went on to say he loved his grandfather, of course.

Tea Tree was his lavender of peace. It was a precious memory of a person, place, and time that changed his whole physiology. He even named the place this happened. This memory would not have surfaced at that moment, if not for a whiff of tea tree with its aromatic charm. Aroma can bring up long forgotten memories. Smell, being personal and individual, travels on the direct olfactory track to our emotional brain. Lots of rewiring can happen here.

Yes, indeed, smell is a potent wizard taking us across thousands of miles and to various places in our lives. It offers many possibilities for healing and for nurturing respites. It can give us peace, call us into action, soothe our aching body, embrace our hurting heart, relieve our grief, and connect us to our dreams.

However, it can also bring up hurt, anger, or tough times. In another class, we were smelling Rose otto. This brought up many lovely responses, and then the man in the back of the class had to pull it away from his nose as tears emerged. Roses in his life meant funerals, and he had recently lost his mother.

In using the sense of smell with a Message, the first step is to choose a soulful aroma to accompany a Message. Enjoy the ones that melt your heart and soothe your soul. This kind of smell ushers in wisdom and love from The Message.

Smell modifies behavior.
It is a powerful trigger for memory and can be used for healing.
Deepak Chopra. MD

Our sense of smell provides a profound inroad to our joy. Joy is certainly a desirable state of being and adds only goodness to the healing process. Those who have lost their sense of smell, called *anosmia*, often suffer from depression, anxiety, and frustration. They have lost the olfactory system's nose-brain connection to our heart, spirit and soul. I have seen joy come back to people when they regain some of their sense of smell. This is sometimes possible.

According to Diane Ackerman in *A Natural History of the Senses*, smell is the first sense that is fully developed at birth. It is how the baby finds its mother, and how the mother finds her baby. This happens right out of the womb of creation and birth. Smell is paramount for survival in many instances. The sense of smell helps the baby find nourishment and nurturing, including the shelter and protection of its mother, father, or guardian.

Pleasant smells can contribute to the well-being of humans.
Aristotle

Aromatic molecules permeate the air and travel up our nose as we breathe. When we find an aroma we love, there is a sense of being home in our inner sanctum. Certain smells tug on our heartstrings and contribute to our sense of well-being. As this personal aroma travels on the breath it helps us accept where we are and provides a way to find some peace moving forward.

Use aromas that bring you peace, touch your soul, invoke joy, and connect you with The Messenger. One of my soul affinities with an aroma took place in 1995 at the International Aromatherapy Conference held at the University of Surrey in Guildford, England. My first whiff of violet leaf (*Viola odorata*) revealed a depth and richness that slowed me down and deepened my breathing. Its strong green leaf odor was a mysterious unfamiliar smell as it brought up the color of green in my mind and embraced the fibers of my being. My mother loved violets and we grew up with them around our home. Violet leaf is a potent, magical wizard of remembrance indeed.

As you inhale your precious aroma, rest with your Message. My personal and professional experiences have shown me that aroma is the silent language of the soul.

Smell is the sense of the imagination.
Jean Jacques Rousseau

Imagine your favorite smells and aromas. Let them take you on your Message's magic carpet ride in search of your golden nuggets with The Messenger as your guide. There are no limits and boundaries as to where it can take you. Be gentle with yourself. Believe in the now and see your future.

For more on smell with essential oils see the chapter, *Essential Oils as Soulful Elements*.

Our Sense of Touch

To touch is to give life.
Michelangelo

Our skin is the largest organ in the body. It surrounds us and protects us. Each of the other five senses have a specific organ location: eyes, nose, mouth, ears. There are many kinds of touch and each involves its own emotional responses. We can be touched physically on the skin, and we can be touched non-physically by seeing or hearing an event that touches our heart.

On a subtle level, there is also the touch of energy. This touch includes the power of the vibration of the spoken word. Then there are times we can feel someone or something around us. There are many forms of touch that serve as powerful healers. Health professionals and therapists are trained in many different modalities of touch for healing and maintaining healthy living.

We usually think of touch as a vehicle that connects us to the world. We usually don't think of it as a way to get in touch with some of the scattered parts of ourselves. By using our sense of touch with a Message, we can put our mind in touch with our heart, increase our heart-mind muscle, and compassionately open ourselves up for more wisdom and insights. Maybe we just relax and enjoy feeling at ease.

Physical touch from another human being is an impressionable exchange. Touch is an urgent sense that gets our attention right away. It takes little effort and has long-lasting effects. I'm reminded of the plane trip where my mother was sitting between me and the man I would be marrying a year later. He and my mother spoke most of the flight, with Mom telling him my life stories. John and I exchanged words only when we were getting off the plane. John told me later that he always remembers how I touched his arm while saying, "Thank you for being so kind to my mother." I didn't remember touching his arm, and there was no agenda attached to this act of kindness. A year later we were married in Naples, Florida, and spent our first married year in Saudi Arabia. Then we came back to Florida to be with Mom until she passed away.

Another powerful memory was with my Touch With Oils® Hand Massage. It developed in the early 1990s while I was using my essential oils blends in retreats and then later with patients in Hospice House. One time at hospice, I was asked if after I finished with Dale, my Wednesday afternoon patient, I would look in on a man in the room down the hall. The man was in and out of consciousness in the bed and very agitated. I waved a little of my blend under Curt's nose and watched his face to be sure it didn't bring up a negative reaction. Then I told him I was going to gently rub his hands, and if he didn't want me to do this, simply squeeze my hand, and I would leave. His tense body started to release and rest. Curt never opened his eyes, and there were no other words. As I finished the method, he was still and calm, so I quietly left.

The next week Curt was motionless and unconscious. I repeated the Touch With Oils® Hand Massage, and while I was on his first hand, he opened his eyes for a few seconds, and said: "You have been here before." The slow gentle rhythmic touch left an imprint and was unconsciously entrained in the emotional part of his brain. Again, I finished and quietly left the room. We repeated this one more time the next week when he was unresponsive, struggling to breath. Later, I learned he passed away a few hours after that time. It was an honor to have been with him.

An act of touch with compassion, gives some relief to struggle and soothes the restless spirit. The following quote is part of the philosophy of my Touch With Oils® Motions of Stillness methods and teachings for nurturing ourselves and nurturing others.

> *Smell and touch are noted to be our most primitive senses.*
> *They are powerful healers when used together with pure integrity.*
> Michelangelo

Touch alone has tremendous impact on our whole being. Touch with smell used with one of The Messages creates a cascading rainbow of possible effects. This environment can touch us in a more enlightened way. The Inner River of Peace is flowing at its best.

Another option to consider is the effects of *tapping* with the Emotional Freedom Technique (EFT). This is a powerful system of tapping designated spots on the body while speaking words of meaning. It can be a *holy habit* way to bring The Message's goodness, peace, and stillness into our whole being. Adding a favorite smell (such as inhaling lemon essential oil from a diffuser) amplifies the effects of the physical and nonphysical entrainment occurring from tapping with smell. Our thoughts, feelings, words, and actions can be changed. Being stuck or frustrated starts to ease up with the wisdom of The Message. *The Tapping Solution*, by Nick Ortner is a worthy read.

Touch is immediate and brings us closer to our inner self. It is easy to create a *holy habit* with our Message doing self-massage on our face, hands or feet, and head or belly (the *hara* or core of our being). Taking a bath or shower is healing in its own right as we get in touch with the water element which makes up a large part of who we are. A calm environment is an invitation for insights to appear. This can happen touching a flower, some water, the earth, or beautiful wooden logs for building a heartwarming fire. These are all times for a pause of stillness.

Touching and rubbing our pets shows us how giving and receiving become one as we give love and receive the nurturing hormone oxytocin. There are many proven comforting health benefits in having an animal to touch. We don't need to talk, and they love us no matter what. Our dog is such a gift to my husband and me. I make time to intentionally rub her belly and ears. Sometimes on my walks, I get an added treat to love on a couple of dogs, a horse, or the three donkeys that come over to the fence for a rub. Embrace the blessings of nature around you.

A touchstone in your pocket is easy and quite comforting. My husband kept a laser pointer in his pocket during his business career. All he did was touch it to remind him all things were possible, and his thoughts shifted instantly. Keep a touchstone with you, and touch it as you repeat a Message, such as: *I am showing up right now and I am holding the vision of a productive business meeting for all those involved.* Now John touches his tiny bottle of jasmine in his pocket.

Touch something of meaning and recite a Message. Take a breath and release any worries, take another breath and slow down, be still, and know simple peace is a possible outcome.

The Messenger is always there with the power to touch us with Spirit. It might be on a gentle breeze or with some raindrops. Just thinking about the Great Holy Spirit coming in on our next few breaths is soothing to our yearning hearts.

Our Sense of Sound

"Music, the perfume of hearing, probably began as a religious act, to arouse groups of people. Drums set the heart sprinting in no time, and a trumpet can transport one on chariots of sound.
As far back as we can see, people made music."
Diane Ackerman, *A Natural History of the Senses*

Humans made sounds long before they spoke words. Animals still make sounds, and some we understand very well. The soulful level of our senses is often expressed with sounds. Sounds can describe somethings better than words can. We hum, sigh, moan, and groan. We say *ahh, umm, ohh* as we take a soulful breath, in and out. Sometimes, when we are too tired or weak to talk, we respond with a sound.

Sounds from instruments have historically been around since human existence. Our hands initially connected with the drum, wooden flutes, and other handmade instruments. We can make them with our hands, and then play them with our hands. Using a Message with a drumbeat resonates to our core. Our Inner River of Peace moves through the core of our being.

Pause for a moment and pull up a memory of a most favorite sound. Where was this? Sounds vibrate through our eardrum into our body. Some sounds take us to a place within where we feel wonderful, such as certain kinds of music, chanting, or nature sounds. There's calming water and ocean sounds, as well as birds and the wind. Nature provides us with sounds of serenity. Slow down here and reflect upon your favorite nature sounds. You can feel the memories.

Sing or hum a song as you go for a walk or sit in the car. Better yet sing The Message to a tune you love. Become a songwriter and honor The Message by writing a song for it. That's what I did back on the Appalachian Trail one time. I still sing this on some of my prayer walks.

Singing or humming a certain sound sends vibrations into our bones and tissue. Prolonged chanting with a word (such as *amen, love, God)* or a sound (such as *om, ah, oh)* vibrates through our body, mind and spirit. Sounds can shift our vibration and change our consciousness. I'm reminded of my memories of the monks' voices, and organ music. There is a sound I call the *Holy Hum* that cannot be described, defined, or confined. It is a soulful sound with a vibrational frequency resonating deeply within us. When we hear it, there is a precious presence. A bit of grace is the rewarding gift.

Listening to our own voice can be very soothing. Try listening to the sound of your recorded voice repeating The Message in a calming way. Use this while moving on a walk, tasting a cup of tea, or coffee, or *Looking at the sky.*

I realized the profound effect of listening to my voice, when I recorded all my notes for an exam on my recorder with Johann Pachelbel's *Canon in D* accompanied with ocean sounds in the background. My hip and nerve pain at the time made it almost impossible to sit and study for more than a few minutes. So, while attending the Sarasota School of Natural Healing Arts, I walked the beautiful beach in Sarasota, Florida, and listened to my voice matching the soothing slow tempo of the music. Just think, I had my feet in the sand, and the surround-sound of the real ocean. The unlimited sight of the sky, along with the smell of the salt breezy air, accompanied this symphony of senses. This became a *holy habit* created out of necessity. I can go back there any time in my imagination. I passed the state and national exam with flying colors.

Certain music, such as classical music like the waltz with a resting heartbeat rhythm, is proven to synchronize our logical left brain with our sensory right brain. The balance of our autonomic nervous system provides a gateway to our Inner River of Peace. Just imagine for a few moments doing this with The Messages. The options are wide open. The results are endless.

Use discernment and protect yourself the best you can from disturbing sounds. Leaf blowers, many noises associated with all kinds of technology, and traffic noises are some that can really scatter our parts. Some noises actually hurt, especially when they jolt us out of a state of harmony. For me, it feels like cruising along smoothly in a car in fourth gear, and suddenly grinding it into first gear. Have you listened to an orchestra tuning up or fingernails scraping the chalkboard? Sounds vibrates through every part of us and can dramatically affect us. Finding our Inner River of Peace restores our sense of well-being.

The most valuable sound chair I know is the invention of Dr. Jeffrey Thompson. Since 1988, he has been doing his magnificent work with the scientific application of sound. As the Founder/Director of his Center for Neuroacoustic Research, he is a physician, musician, composer, inventor, educator, and author of the highest order. He gathers sounds such as nature, NASA's space recordings, and his own musical compositions for each level of brain wave entrainment. He invented an advanced system of finding the frequency of each person's individual *keynote* to bring the autonomic nervous system into harmony. When I experienced this with him, he recorded my voice humming *the key of me* after he played it on a keyboard. I felt like I was home. Then placing my hum in the background, he created compositions for each healing level of sound frequency. The sound chair he invented works with my CDs in the key of me. This has been a major *holy habit* in my health regime. When my husband and I lived with our dog for a year in our RV, while still working our essential oil company, we took out the chairs and put in our sound chair. This was profound, fun, and wonderful.

    Sounds are all around us. Sometimes, we are more aware of the sounds, when we hear the pauses and gaps between sounds. Notice how sounds make you feel. Be conscious of the ones that make you feel wonderful, and others not so wonderful. Note the sounds and places that inspire you and bring more of them into your life. *Anchor way down deep* (from Message Four) in sounds that soothe your soul. Then you are in a silent place to observe the waves of life and know that they too shall pass and dissipate.

Our Sense of Taste

Our heads are so often in another place
that we don't really taste what we are eating.
Clyde Reid, *Celebrate the Temporary*

The delicious, delectable delights of tasting our favorite foods are part of the real joys of life. However, it appears that many times we have lost touch with being conscious of what we are eating and how it tastes.

Our tasting times are some of our most social times. The four main category of tastes are sweet, salt, sour, and bitter. They each have their own receptor sites on different areas of our tongue. Food is a huge source of pleasure and friendship, which accounts for its presence at most social events. Rarely do humans choose to eat in solitude or silence, although it can be lovely. Celebrations of all kinds, rewards, meetings, and gatherings on all levels include food and drink. The tasting connections we share together are also a bonding experience. Many senses overlap here. Breaking bread together supports the need for community. The touch of a handshake or hug, aromas and tastes, and sounds of voices and laughter, all contribute to the joys of life.

Create a quiet time when you are eating and make it a momentary break from your activities. There is a space here to call in a Message just to remind you to be conscious. See what this is like. Taste is reported to be as much as 70-80% smell. When we are under the weather with congestion and a cold, we lose our ability to taste our food. This makes us feel even worse. Taste and smell are stars in the palette of our senses. They remind us of special occasions and times we have shared with others. They are hard-wired memories for holidays like Thanksgiving or Christmas. Taste and smell go together, and the memory brings up a vision.

> *The truth about vanilla is that it's as much a smell as a taste.*
> Diane Ackerman, *A Natural History of the Senses*

Smell vanilla and you can taste it. Taste vanilla and you can smell it. Vanilla is one of the most cherished tastes and smells. It is luscious, delicious, and boosts our moods.

Two of the most universal and historically enjoyed delights to our taste buds are chocolate and vanilla. They are feel-good flavors and fragrances that soothe and nurture our whole being. Chocolate and vanilla often bring up a soulful sound, like *umm, ohhh, ahhh*. They add their richness to many of our foods and drinks, and create strong memories with visons, thoughts, and emotions. Have a piece of chocolate and recite your Message. If this becomes a *holy habit*, the entrainment of one to the other is inevitable. When you eat chocolate, you'll think of The Message. When you recite The Message, you will think of chocolate. *Holy habits* are to be healing games and good medicine.

When I passed around smelling-sticks in my classes, charged with a few drops of pure peppermint essential oil, people had yummy nose-brain responses. Peppermint brought up instantaneous memories of Christmas and candies. Sage and spices often brought up Thanksgiving, and orange brought up Dreamsicles and sweets. All these smells are connected to tastes. Often someone says they taste a smell in the back of their throat, and all they had was a few whiffs of the smelling stick. The Olfactory Research Institute did a study on men's favorite smells. The top two were lavender and pumpkin pie. I smiled. Yes indeed, lavender for mental stress, and pumpkin pie to soothe the belly.

In modern days of multitasking and complexity, often we drink our aromatic coffee, and eat snacks or meals while watching television, standing and gulping, driving, working, talking on the phone, or using a concoction of other devices. Our digestive system says: *Hey, what are you doing up there in the head? I'm down here working hard to digest and make healthy use of what you are sending down to me, and you can't even give me the dignity to pay some attention to me? I need all that energy you are burning up elsewhere to help out with digestion in my department.*

Our body and digestive tract deserve our full attention. Our immune system depends on a healthy gut, as does our brain. Can you remember eating a piece of chocolate or a favorite food that made you pause with a sound and sigh like *yumm, ahhh*. This pleasant emotional response gets recorded in your cells with the positive corresponding brain chemistry.

Experiment in baby steps. Try sitting down each time you eat something. Notice what you're eating, how it tastes, and how you feel. The command we give our dog, Muga, is *sit down*, before she gets her meal or treat. Why shouldn't we do the same? Simply *sit down*. One slow breath is a good idea, too.

Try combining a favorite food, coffee, and tea with a Message. Savor the flavor and the full experience of all this swirling pleasure. Give it your full attention and notice what happens in your heart's brain. Your heart-mind muscle will get activated as well. Let's face it, we all love food. Some of our favorites can also be extremely healthy. This serves us well in many ways. It creates the time and space for our Inner River of Peace to flow with ease, and for us to feel a touch of joy.

Delicious, delightful, and delectable are three of my favorite words for a wonderful meal. Bring back the *holy habit* way of eating a meal or teatime in your life. The brain in our belly says: slow down, be still, and cherish simple feel-good moments. There is contentment and happiness to be found here.

The value of teatime was an eye-opening experience for me. I spent a college summer studying abroad with one month

Power of the 5 Senses Plus 2

in England learning English History and Shakespeare. When I experienced my first real teatime in mid-afternoon, I thought: *Wow, this is lovely. What are we missing in our fast-dashing society?* Ever since then I have loved and valued this special time of regeneration. It's a time of embracing our senses and contemplating (even for a few seconds) the beauty of one or more of The Messages of Universal Truth. When we are completely present and appreciative, it becomes a window to our heart-mind muscle and Inner River of Peace. It's a little respite for a mental vacation and a little happy sustenance. Our lives don't honor this time very much; however, we can claim it every chance we get.

There are lots of options for special times involving taste in which we can really decide to be fully present. Find one that works for you and embrace it. Decide to enjoy these moments whenever you can, wherever you are.

Our Sense of Sight

The human eye adores gazing. The eye is always drawn to the shape of a thing. It finds deep consolation and sense of home in special shapes. Deep within the human mind, there is a fascination with the circle because it satisfies some longing within us. It is one of the most universal and ancient shapes in the universe.

John Donahue, *Anam Cara*

We are bombarded with sights and sounds. There is no shortage of sights or sounds in the material world and on our devices. Crowds of traffic, buildings, and people give us a certain feeling. Then there is the beach, forest, desert, mountains, valleys, meadows, and sweet little gardens. We can pull up and create any thing that we would like to see with our inner sight of vision and imagination.

Pieces of art often bring contemplative pauses. Sights can transport us to another time and place. They let us disengage for a time and a rest. The National Gallery of Art in Washington, D.C. does this for me. Living nearby as a child, I loved going there. The huge building is awesomely beautiful.

The hallways, fountains, statues, and masterful art of the ages, transports me to an inner place I love. As an adult, I realize this inner place is my Inner River of Peace.

Observe how it feels to see things with a loving eye. Our natural world is full of rich colors with glorious rainbows, sunrises, sunsets, and flowers. These are exceptional sites to bring in the wisdom and love of The Messages. My mother loved looking at the clouds and seeing what figures they showed her. This was very peaceful for her. I now look at the clouds and think of Mom. Light sparkling on the leaves of trees, children and puppies playing, a beautiful ballet, or an amazing orchestra are some other sights that can touch our soul.

I have a grateful memory of the time my family took a huge trip in a motor home across the country from Washington, D.C. to California when I was in ninth grade. We were standing in the center of a busy San Francisco street waiting for the trolley. Looking over at a park, I saw a man moving very slowly and deliberately with his arms and legs. The sight of him pulled me in and made me pause. *What is he doing? Whatever that is, I am a part of that.* It was not until age forty-one, that I started tai chi lessons from a master. After a major surgery, it was time to shift away from high impact aerobics and heavy weightlifting. I opened the *Naples Daily Newspaper,* and there was the face of a man that just moved to Naples offering tai chi classes. The sight in the park that day made such an impression on me; the feeling of stillness remains. Dreams come true in a timing of their own. Hold onto your dreams as The Messages guide you.

Dawn and dust display an amazing color and light show for the eyes. This is a beautiful time of transition to visit a Message. Night shifts into day, and then the yang light of day shifts to the yin darkness of night. It is also a window of time to receive some of our best information from The Messages. The Messenger comes in. These two times of the day are when the veil between the visible and invisible world is the thinnest. For many of us these two times of day call and draw us like a magnet. The heart yearns for these times of stillness, rest and peace. Our innate connection and love for nature becomes visible. The amber glow and the light are spiritual nutrition.

Do your best not to get bombarded and thrown off center with constant visual stimulus that disturbs the central nervous system. We live in a world that can get wildly visual. Faster, bigger, and more does not mean better. Computers, phones and other devices, along with television screens influence every cell of our body, with significant effects on our whole being. Notice what you are watching when you feel irritated or jumpy, and what makes you feel good. It's as simple as that.

Honor comforting sights that you really enjoy. Bring as many as you can into your life. When was the last time you laid on your back and used your eyes to gaze at the sky?

Our Plus Two Senses
Our Sense of Movement

Harmonious and efficient movement prevents wear and tear.
More important, however, is what it does to the image of ourselves and
our relationship to the world around us.
Moshe Feldenkris, D. Sc.

The body was made to move, and moving the body gives us a fluid sense of freedom. It helps ground us as it serves as a temple for the soul, and yet also a chemistry tube constantly striving for homeostasis. It is also a space suit that protects us, and a car that takes us places and needs to be driven. Movement transmits energy and flushes out accumulated stresses. If we move the body every day, we can wash the chalkboard clean of daily accumulated dross. Daily clean-up makes for a better next day.

Some of the other senses involve movement in our invisible mind field such as smell (breathing), sights (seeing), and sounds (listening). Some also involve more physical movements like touch (physical) and taste (eating and drinking). They all involve movement on some level within us.

Moving the body exercises joints, muscles, and connective tissue, while improving circulation and increasing oxygen to the brain. It moves emotions through the body, so they don't get stuck and cause trouble. Movement has always been a part of daily life. However, with more technology and modern life, there is a decrease in the amount of physical movement we give our bodies. Our body wants us to take it for a walk.

Everything in nature reminds us to move and reminds us to rest. We see moving waters and changing winds. We see floating clouds and swaying trees. Then there comes a time for still waters, settled wind, clear skies, and strong-stellar grandmother trees. We are part of nature and our well-being depends on moving, changing, floating, and swaying. There is a time to be still and know; there is a time to take action and go.

One day at the beach, I was in one of my gazing times, and a group of seven pelicans showed up and flew in circles of formation over my head. They flapped their large graceful wings to move when it was time to take action. When it was time to rest and restore their energy, they became motions of stillness as they glided along the top of the waves. The pelicans showed me: we must flap and flow in life. Move and rest; act and wait. Each is dependent upon the other. This offering of pelican wisdom brought such peace. Don't forget to give your eyes a little gazing time.

When you go outside, just move the body and notice the condition of the sky, the wind, and the light. Breathe and disengage from the world for a few deep breaths. Repeat one of The Messages and allow yourself to merge with *your* Inner River of Peace.

Dance is a universal, cross-cultural way of moving. All cultures dance to engage in life and celebrations. Look at the increase in dance lessons and classes in these modern times. Dance is coupled with sounds, music, drums, and all types of instruments. Dance with a Message and dream your world of harmony into being. Release the dross, and dance into *your* Inner River of Peace the very best that you can. Just move the body.

Power of the 5 Senses Plus 2

There are many professional movement therapies that show us our Inner River of Peace. These are more popular than ever, which indicates again the need to move in these times of less moving. The Feldenkrais Method® of physical structural awareness with movement is really coming into its own. Moshe Feldenkrais, who passed away in the 1980s, was before his time in proclaiming the theory that moving the body in different ways also increases neuroplasticity in the brain.

Our spirit and soul want to move. Some ways serve as meditations, such as, tai chi, qigong, yoga, prayer walking, running, and biking. The right kind of movement lifts our spirit and gives us the feeling of freedom. What is your right kind of movement?

Tai Chi is a gentle yet powerful form of moving the body. In my private tai chi lessons, we spent months on a qigong routine. Each week we first rubbed a drop of Frankincense in our palms. My teacher said he never had anything activate his Qi (life force energy) so quickly. Looking in the mirror, I saw our hands moving in golden gloves. Because I made the choice to *Show Up and Hold the Vision* for a focused qigong lesson, the gentle power of this practice came forth. Moving the body, with smell and a Message is pleasantly unforgettable.

It's important to move in a way that is enjoyable to you, not a dreaded chore that has to be done at the health club. Happy thoughts and feelings create happy cells and tissue; and happy words and actions will follow. Learning something new is great for the mind and body. Discernment and wisdom are the call. If it brings you peace, you are in your river.

Edith Hall in her book, *Aristotle's Way*, reports Aristotle's philosophy in his school of thought was based on *peripateo*. In Greek it translates as *I go for a walk*. He believed that having experiences was the way to a balanced and healthy life in living one's purpose.

This was part of his theory on finding happiness.

The first form of prayer was walking in a circle. No wonder we love to walk; it resonates in our being. Many sages, thinkers, and writers are known to have walked for inspiration, intuition, and imagination. It's a contemplative time. Sometimes, we think better while moving. Moving starts the thinking-engine.

Walking alone silently is a lovely form of prayer. Walking with a friend in conversation is also one of my favorite things. Our bodies were not made to sit for long periods of time. Our hips, legs, and back agree. We don't need a research study to know this.

Bring to mind a meaningful walking experience in your life. It might simply be strolling with a loved one holding hands. Wandering through a beautiful place in nature is always a heartfelt gem. It can also be walking down the streets of New York City, if your heart-mind muscle is in gear. I recall a wonderful experience while walking through the hustle and bustle of NYC and then walking into St Patrick's Cathedral. There was only one other person there. The stillness and silence were beautiful. Our Inner River of Peace travels with us, so it can come through anywhere.

In one of the transformational times of my life, I had an *aha* moment realizing exercise heals a broken spirit. After losing the ownership of a tennis club and all it involved, I had moved from a profession that was mainly movement outdoors to a mostly sedentary indoor profession in real estate. I was like a restless dog that needed exercise. I joined a health club with the purpose to exercise and release my frustration and monkey mind. Early on, I noticed it was really lifting my spirits. We think of exercise for physical health, meanwhile the brain is releasing new chemicals that lift the spirit. All of a sudden, we are feeling pretty good about ourselves.

Movement of the right kind, at the right time, in the different seasons of life are good medicine for self-esteem. Moving with a Message lifts the spirit and soothes the soul. The horse with a broken spirit can come alive again.

When I feel stuck, I get up and move around or go outside. I go for a walk. I breathe differently and I feel better. I get clarity on what's going on and what's next. It might even just be that it's time to rest. Sometimes, I do the tai chi slow walk while reading, or talking on the phone.

Go for a walk with one of The Messages and notice how many senses you can experience. There is powerful wisdom in our body. Move and listen. Our spirit dances and touches the soul. May we all honor our path, support the wholeness and holy-ness of our being, and love who we are every step of the way.

Our future is being created by each day we live.

Movement opens the channels and space for our intuition and imagination to flow. This provides a time to rest from the engagement in the world. The Messenger speaks to us here.

Our Senses of Intuition and Imagination

Intuition and Imagination go beyond the normal range of the five senses. Each of these two words serves each other and inspires the other to appear. Both guide us and give us insights on how to be more of all we can be. Intuition and imagination provide a form of nutrition to our ways of thinking. We get outside the fixed framework of our minds. They can affect or be affected by the other senses. Having them converge is an opening to the invisible world of prayer, meditation, and moments of stillness.

Our intuition and imagination remind us of our dreams, lead us into following them, and assist us in finding our raison d'etre. Together or separately, they show us the beautiful power of deep rest and silence. The Inner River of Peace flows. It is a fluid experience of a touch of grace.

Intuition and imagination connect us to inspiration and invention. Inventions start with these senses in heart and mind of something we want or need. Albert Einstein is reported to have said imagination is more important than knowledge. The insights available to us are especially wonderful if they find us doing our part to bring about what we are imagining and dreaming. To be purposely inventing ourselves, throughout our life, is a heroic journey of discovery. The rewards are unknown unless we go there.

Intuition and Imagination shift our awareness in the moment. We think differently. We observe. We heal. They are portals into our Inner River of Peace. Wisdom and love abound here. As we think and feel differently, our words and actions change. We start to live more in harmony with all our parts. The travels into our future are enriched and inspirational.

With your heart-mind muscle, see if you can recall a time in life when this kind of harmony happened for you in any way. It lifts the spirit just to think about it. This is something you can visualize. You can imagine yourself there again. Your intuition will guide you. It is our silent and invisible compass.

If we don't move the body, our muscles fade away. If we don't use our intuition and imagination, they fade away, too. Give your wonderful self some time to cherish all your senses by simply inviting them in and noticing how they serve you.

Intuition

"Quick perception of truth without conscious attention or reasoning, knowledge from within, instinctive knowledge or feeling, an immediate knowledge, or envisagement of an object."
Funk & Wagnalls New College Standard Dictionary

The other senses mentioned before can ignite the inner wisdom of our intuition. When you ask your intuition for help, it will show up with guidance and insights when least expected. They are often *Aha* moments with a capital A. Be curious and open to this part of your consciousness, and let it grow into a greater presence in your life. Intuition arrives in an instant as a surprise visitor. The more we appreciate it, the more it shows up, and the better we get at partnering with our intuition.

Quiet times of prayer, meditation, contemplation, and reflection are all invitations to our intuition. Being silent in this way can sometimes be interpreted as doing nothing. What looks like doing nothing here is being everything. This is where we find out what is really going on, and what we need to know. It can even correct our course in an instant if necessary.

Take the time to show up for yourself and hold the vision for clarity, guidance, and the love of the Highest. Each Message holds this goodness within, waiting to be delivered in divine timing. These mysteries and surprises are refreshing gifts in life. They give us hope and present the opportunity to build our faith.

The real challenge, in a world overflowing with outward noise and rushing rivers of information, is to really trust our intuition. We tend to doubt it, worry if we even have any, and question its truth when it arrives. The more we ask for it and practice trusting it, the stronger the heart-mind muscle becomes with its amazing ability to work (love made visible) together. Sometimes, this takes me to my knees and tears trickle down.

Start with small steps and build your trust in your inner wisdom. Keeping The Messages with you is one way to do this. It is especially important to recognize the wisdom with some form of gratification. It is always a beautiful two-way street when giving and receiving with integrity become one.

Our culture has trained us so well to live in our intellect that we have literally lost touch with our senses. We simply do not hear the messages. We do not listen to the wisdom of our body, the guidance of our intuition.
Clyde Reid, *Celebrate the Temporary*

We recognize our intuition when there is an unquestionable realization it is the truth. There is often a sense of peace, because a decision has been made for us, even if it calls for lots of courage. The more we do this, the more our trust grows with experience and awareness. Faith is the ground we stand on, even when it seems like no ground is there.

> *Whenever you Think you are limited,*
> *Look at the sky.*   Message Two

Embracing our intuition creates a spark to ignite the wisdom and love from The Messages to appear. Remember to look up with a heart full of thanksgiving.

Imagination

> *Thou will keep him in perfect peace when*
> *imagination is stayed on thee.*
> Isaiah, xxxv.3

Our Imagination is a very powerful part of our entire being. How we imagine something in our mind's eye, feel it in our gut, and power it up in our will center - eventually determines our behavior. This is a highly creative aspect of our abilities to get answers and give birth to ideas. We imagine, we actively participate in some way, and we create it. We see it, we feel it, and we take action. Divine timing and order are in this mix of energies. Sometimes the call is simply to wait, while we hang onto imagining our desired outcome.

Our imagination can be an inner journey of our dreams, desires, and discoveries. It can also be an outer journey into the quantum field of potentiality. All these visions awaken our spirit and set it free to fly on the wings of hope. Use your imagination to visualize possible new thoughts and feelings with The Messages. The deeper the connection, the more The Messages become part of your newly expanded ways of thinking and feeling.

Here are a few quotes to inspire your heart to think and your mind to feel in some other new ways.

Imagination is the star in man, the celestial and super-celestial body.
Martin Ruland

Imagination is therefore a concentrated extract of the life forces, both physical and psychic.
C.J. Jung

Where does your imagination go when it gets a chance to wander? Daydreaming is a valued element of creation and problem solving. Go back to a time/place/event when your imagination was creating something wonderful and visualize the sensations you experienced. Was there a presence of peace? Notice how instantly thoughts, feelings, and memories around this rise to the surface of your consciousness. This can be a good place to revisit now and then.

Use your senses to enhance each Message's meaning for you. From here we can function in our life from a higher level, experiencing more joy and feeling more love, first for our self and then for each other. Through osmosis, this affects those in our environment. Be still and notice when this happens. It's miraculous.

If you can see it, the body can feel it. The body doesn't know the difference between what is real and what is visualized and imagined. Have you ever had a dream that was so real, your body was physically reacting to it? The physical reaction can be so extreme that you are awakened.

One time when this happened to me, the dream was so emotionally painful that my body was physically experiencing the pain in the dream. I awakened in the midst of the pain, and my body was still in the same pain. I felt completely out of sorts. I was home alone with the dog, so I got up, kept walking around to relieve the pain, and then called my sister in the middle of the night to talk. Praise God for best friend sisters. Eventually, I realized the pain was the result of what was happening in my dream, which was also part of the rest of my life.

The power of the mind is not to be taken lightly. It is to be honored and used for our good, even when it is showing us a tough challenge. This is all the more reason to be focused on being in our Inner River of Peace as much as possible.

Our senses and imagination with any of The Messages, act like a magnet. This pulls in all the little filaments of wisdom and love from the universe through The Message to serve us well. Truth and goodness abound, as *your* Inner River of Peace comes to light.

Use your imagination to visualize the *Love Rainbow of Trust* that I describe in my personal story with Message Eight. Take a quick re-read. Imagine what your rainbow looks like. Decide you are going to live on it and walk its walk. When we fall off, we can climb back on the next day.

> *You must Trust me like never before,*
> *if you want to survive.*   *Message Eight*

Our intuition and imagination are key senses that give us clarity in our life. They help us adjust our thinking. Thinking in a new way is a breath of fresh air, a sense of freedom and self-control is regained. When our thinking changes, so do our feelings, then comes the news words and actions.

> *The world we have created is a process of our thinking;*
> *it cannot be changed without changing our thinking.*
> Albert Einstein

This starts with changing our inner world. Here we find the guiding stars of our intuition and imagination waiting for us. The

Messenger walks before you, by your side and behind you, above you, below you and within you. *Your* Inner River of Peace and the gentle power of the wisdom in the Ten Messages of Love are pillars of strength waiting to embrace us. Know you are getting in touch with the power of love that runs deeply within you. Tapping into this deeply *seeded* powerful Source as often as possible is the purpose and inspiration for this book.

Be gentle with yourself.

You are your own gemstone to be celebrated.

You and your life are precious.

Summary

Our sensory perceptions overlap, intertwine, and swirl with our thoughts and emotions. They serve as links to the Inner River of Peace within all of us. Thus, they share the same mission as The Messages. The wisdom and love can be visible, such as when it comes through or materializes in physical forms like a person or event. They also are invisible, such as the sense of peace that everything is going to be okay somehow on some level, even if we can't see it right now. It's all part of the program called human life. It is a most adventuresome challenge, offering golden nuggets and diamonds along the way.

If you wish to work toward celebrating the temporary with your whole self, then three things are necessary. All three are incredibly simple. One is relaxing. The second is breathing. And the third is depriving yourself by turning off the sound of your voice in order to allow your senses to emerge.
Clyde Reid, *Celebrate the Temporary*

Let's come to our senses with awareness and appreciation for how they inspire us to create, stimulate us to move, and soothe our weary bones. Then there is the delicious joy they bring to our lives.

Creating *holy habits* with The Messages and our senses help us explore, remember, and restore different parts of us that are out of sorts. The power of the senses provides a gateway to our Inner River of Peace. In this place of peace and harmony, we find compassion, wisdom, and love. When we find this within ourselves, then we have this to offer to others.

All our senses have a direct impact on our autonomic nervous system. This comes out of the core of our emotional brain. The energy that creates fight or flight, also creates rest and restoration. These are unconscious responses that instantly happen from sensory stimuli. Using our senses as we *Focus on the Light and Love* in our life, enriches The Messages.

Explore the ideas and try some simple ways to use the power of the senses to empower The Message. Treat your cellular responses to some peace and harmony. These are healing games and good medicine for our immune system, nervous system, endocrine system, and all the rest of our systems. The brain chemistry shifts, the heart pumps accordingly, and we move into a better place.

The different senses might remind you of certain Messages, and The Messages can remind us of certain senses. Simply reading The Message might bring up a memory. For example, perhaps Message Ten about love might remind you of roses or bring up the thought of a color. Perhaps Message Four about *Anchor way down deep* brings up a color like green or blue, or the memory of a wonderful sailboat ride. See if any of The Messages bring to mind a smell, a sight, or a sound.

Embrace each Message of universal truth and honor it with loving attention by spending some time there. There is goodness here. Celebrate who you are with your senses and allow them to be enlightening partners. You are the only person who knows what this wisdom and love is for you.

Remember: Stop, Look, and Listen (SLL) to what is really going on. Honor *Slow, Still, and Simple (SSS)* in your day and your life any way you can. Even one little action is enough to start the momentum to shift. This is part of *your* Inner River of Peace adventure. Be full-of-thanks all along the way. Perhaps today can be your favorite day, even if it's just in your imagination. Magnificent things happen from the imaginative genius part of us coupled with the Grace of God.

*Twenty years from now you will be more disappointed by the things
you didn't do than by the ones you did do.
So throw off the bowlines. Sail away from the safe harbor.
Catch the trade winds in your sails.
Explore. Dream. Discover.*
Attributed to Mark Twain

Relate this to what works for you right now. Explore, Dream, and Discover are inspirational words speaking to each of us in our own way. It's not about being reckless with a knee-jerk decision; it's about standing in the truth of our Self. With our unique gifts, we can courageously follow this guidance as we carry forth on the heroic expedition of our life.

The above quote is on the *Welcome to Port of Mount Dora* placard by the lighthouse in Mount Dora, Florida. My husband, doggie Muga, and I take walks here often, and we read The Message together. This is one of our favorite quotes because it lifts our spirits and inspires us to hang onto our heart of the explorer archetype, no matter our age, situation, or location.

My prayer for you to imagine:

*Dear God,
Increase my awareness to hear your Guidance
Give me the Courage to follow it when I hear it.
Let me do this with the kind of Faith that moves mountains.
Amen*

This prayer came in when a circle of dear precious friends blessed my Oil Lady Aromatherapy® shop-studio in a ceremonial opening in 1997 in Naples, Florida. This giant leap of faith was moving my business from my home to a business out on the street.

The prayer is about giving up and releasing our self-doubts and worries. It's about stepping out in trust when our intuition shows us the way. The financial numbers made no common sense that favored me signing a rental lease. I knew down deep inside I was going to do it anyway. It was the call, and it was about trusting my intuitional pull. The call along with my intuition that day was stronger and more loving than any of the voices in my head. Thank goodness.

We had nine wonderful years there. To this day the above prayer is still one of my main prayers. Maybe it can be one of yours, too.

Essential Oils as Soulful Elements

An essential oil, the bonding medium for the soul of the plant, is uniquely suited to act as the physical entity that can facilitate an interface between plant and human souls.

Rudolph Steiner

Each of us is a one-of-a-kind soulful element. When soulful elements recognize each other, there is an innate response that opens our heart and calls in our spirit. Here lives our Inner River of Peace. From this place of compassion, we are able to connect to the Inner River of Peace in others. Ultimately, we move into a remembrance where we hold a reverence for nature and life in all things great and small.

Nature abounds with soulful elements of all kinds. At times we are drawn to fire, water, wind, and earth. Sunrises, sunsets, water, mountains, forests, and deserts seem to magnetically attract us. Sometimes, it's just gazing out the window, looking up at the sky, or putting our back up against a tree. When we experience other soulful elements, there is a feeling of being home. This can happen with our pets, our gardens, wonderful foods made with love, and the aroma of a genuine essential oil. These are gateways to our Inner River of Peace.

Nature gives us her most precious liquid in essential oils to nurture us through life. They are extracted, mainly through distillation, from various parts of plants and trees. Most essential oils exist in glands or sacs within plant structures, such as leaves and flowers. Before the discovery of fire and invention of distillation, they were gathered simply by cutting and squeezing parts of plants and trees. They also placed leaves in a bowl of water, made from stones in the ground. They waited for the blazing sun to burst the oil glands. When you crush a peppermint leaf in your fingers, the sac bursts open and you smell peppermint. When you pop the sac in an orange rind, it burns your lips.

From the very first time I came into contact with essential oils, I realized they were soulful elements with a royal mission to serve, assist, and protect us humans in many ways on many levels, on our travels through life. They also remind us to celebrate life and who we soulfully are, as they connect us to our Inner River of Peace. They have the ability to remind us of our dreams. The wisdom and love they have for us abounds.

Essential Oils as Soulful Elements

Matter is most spiritual in the perfume of plants.
Rudolph Steiner

Essential oils were among the origins of medicine, due to the medicinal natural chemical constituents in their liquid. They were also the original perfumes due to their aromas. If you are drawn to the powerful aromas of authentic essential oils, then I lovingly embrace the idea of you using them with each Message.

The bonding ability essential oils have with The Message's wisdom and love, creates a nose-brain-body entrainment that takes no effort and needs no words. Breathe them into your brain and lungs with The Message. Use the Simple Focused-Breathing Technique described at the end of each chapter in *Contemplative Moments.* Thus, we create new *holy habits*, with holy substances, honoring the soulful Inner River of Peace within us.

We will briefly explore essential oils as microcosms of holistic medicine, delivering their unique medicine and message for each of us. Then we'll reveal their Royal Mission in the power of threes. The ten essential oils presented here as some top choices, based on my personal and professional experiences since 1989. The purpose is to continually create new *holy habits* that keep us in the flow of our Inner River of Peace.

Before the review at the end of this chapter, we will cover safe use. This encompasses honoring the essential oils as Mother

Nature's most precious gifts to us. We are called to preserve the earth's supply of essential oils and be good stewards of the lands. Our reward is the return to our Inner River of Peace and our innate relationship with Nature. Our whole sense of well-being is enriched and regenerated.

My Personal Story

The first-time essential oils came into my life was in 1989. I had never heard of essential oils or aromatherapy before then. I was on a searching mission to restore my health. This involved six years of visiting fifteen doctors and having three surgeries. My mission was to figure out how to resolve my health challenges. This involved lots of exploration and faith on my part. Not trying and not believing in possibilities was not an option. With faith and trust, I kept moving through doors as I found each one open.

I lived with physical pain in varying degrees for those six years with a nerve and cyst playing against each other, a frozen shoulder, extreme headaches, and thyroid issues. My marriage was ending, and my father's Alzheimer's was progressing. This created physical and emotional exhaustion, constant pain, and very little

Essential Oils as Soulful Elements

sleep. It was a journey I had to go on to get to where I was supposed to be. I went out searching, and it took a buffet table of healing games and good medicine to get me there. This included six months of training at the Sarasota School of Natural Healing Arts in Florida.

It was my first aromatherapy massage from an English therapist that turned my life around. A new world opened up to me. I have always been very sensitive to smell. Perfumes were overpowering. Why was I more than fine and feeling a tremendous sense of peace and comfort with these smells? What are these essential oils and what is aromatherapy? They connected me to my Inner River of Peace instantly. I realized whatever this was, some part of me already knew it and was born to be with it. It reminded me of the river of love I felt coursing through my veins as a little child. I went up to the beach that evening and tears trickled down. There was something beautiful here that I had to follow. My spirit was lifting me up as I dreamed, explored and discovered a whole new world that made my heart very happy.

So, the next season of my life began. I didn't know how it would play out. This was the true work I prayed for and needed. Compassionate work I was passionate about.

Work is love made visible.
Kahlil Gibran

When we have pain, our soul is trying to get our attention. The soul speaks to us through the body. If we don't get The Message right away, our soul will get our attention, one way or another. Pain is here to take us somewhere. Follow the pain and keep searching for relief. Keep trying things that seem authentic to you. When you get in *your* Inner River of Peace, the river takes you. I trained in England like I was going to the grocery store. There was no jet lag. Purdue University and several amazing teachers showed up also. I realized the money I had saved in my previous work was for education in this work.

My personal and professional life with essential oils has shown me the wisdom and the love they carry. This comes from practical physical experience and nonphysical insights. The truth is the two cannot be separated, which is the very nature of essential oils. They do not allow the separation of our physical healing from our nonphysical healing. Essential oils provide powerful assistance to the universal Messages of Love.

While working with my clients and customers, essential oils showed me their capacity to bring relief to the hurting body and peace to the scattered mind. They can open our heart and call in our spirit. They can also show us the way to follow our life-path dreams and have been known to give us the courage to act. They have divine timing for each person's needs in each season of life.

Divine order and divine grace inspire us to take the next step in creating our future.

Essential oils do what they need to do for each person. I heard one time: *Just get us there, and we'll do the work. We need you as the vessel to get us there.* This came in when I was taking some of my blends to my dad who had cracked his ribs. He was in pain and asked if I thought the oils could help. I said I wasn't sure, but let's try it. He was amazed at the pain relief and the comfort. I smiled thinking about the essential oils on their soulful mission for my father. Essential oils became my personal partners on a new level.

While teaching my first classes around my kitchen table, I realized humans have always used essential oils throughout history for the same reasons: to anoint, cleanse, communicate, purify, and protect. Each of these words has many meanings on physical and nonphysical levels. We use modern ways to do ancient things, for the same reasons.

The methods of use are changed to suit the culture. When I was in Ecuador and Peru, the medicine people put floral water in their mouths and spit-sprayed it on the person they were healing. I smiled and thought how amazing. I'm making Lavender Mist in a bottle and misting people to wash away the dross of the moment and lift their spirit. Spitting wouldn't work in our society today.

Misting works just fine and the effects are profound. Misting is an excellent, simple way to enhance each of The Messages.

Essential oils have been making a slow and solid comeback since their re-discovery in the early 1900s. Our current times of complexity and noise find humans and the earth spread thin. The stress on humans and the stress on the earth coincide. There are more people on the planet than ever before. This means there are more ways to thrive and more ways not to thrive. Essential oils are sorely needed as part of the restoration of health for humans and the earth. This includes the rejuvenation of their reverent relationship. If we look at the state of humans, we see the same state of the earth. If we want to know the state of the earth, look at the state of humans.

Our survival depends upon our connection with the earth, and our compassion for each other. Essential oils have a Royal Mission to restore a harmonic convergence between humans and nature. It starts at home with each of us caring for ourselves. The musical notes of essential oils make up the orchestra of soulful elements and our Inner River of Peace provides the anchor. All this is needed to keep the vessel (us) afloat.

Essential Oils as Microcosms of Holistic Medicine

Essential oils are in the forefront of Integrative Functional Medicine. The earth can barely keep up with the worldwide increasing demand and consumption that is spreading like a wildfire. The reason for this resurgence of interest in essential oils is attributed to the power and comfort of their natural medicinal chemical constituents and the instantaneous responses from their aromas. Our many parts are treated holistically. Our heart opens, and our spirit flows in our Inner River of Peace.

The Ten Messages of Love with essential oils serve each other well. They meet in their joint royal mission for connecting humans with their Inner River of Peace. They strengthen our heart-mind muscle and touch our soul with their beauty, wholeness, and holy-ness.

There are two top attributes of aromatherapy. First, they have the ability to instantaneously relieve stress, whether it's short-term anxiety or long-term chronic stress. Secondly, they support and create a healthier immune system, short-term colds or long-term immune issues. The key is safe use of the right essential oil, in the right dilution and method of delivery, for the right length of time.

Essential oils are cross-cultural without concern for age, gender, condition, or location. They transcend time and place. My times with the women of Saudi Arabia, Inca men and women in the Andes, and unconscious people in Hospice House, showed me this gentle power. Essential oils are here to remind us of the oneness within all of us creatures great and small. Throughout history, as soon as humans were on the planet, essential oils were part of survival and celebration. The connection of humans and nature is a symbiotic relationship to be cherished.

Forgotten and ignored for many years, aromatic essences are coming back into their own, for any researchers and for a large section of the public opinion, as stars of medicine. Even at present we nevertheless possess, in aromatherapy, a priceless tool.
Jean Valnet, MD

Essential oils as highly concentrated volatile liquids serving as physical medicine and emotional medicine, just by being who they are. Each works unto the other. Their extremely high electromagnetic frequencies come into play as well. They work through the air that we stand in and breathe. Osmosis is silent, simple, and profound.

The **physical liquid** of essential oils, with all its medicinal properties, works on the physical body, such as lavender's anti-inflammatory properties relieving painful burns on unbroken skin. Blends used in massage relieves tight tissue and sore muscles. Some essential oils used safely in steam tents relieve congestion (in body and mind) and sinus pain, due to antibacterial, antiviral, decongestant properties, and much more.

This liquid happens to have the purest and most powerful healthy aroma on earth. The **nonphysical aromatic vapors** travel through our nose to the olfactory bulb. They lock into olfactory neurons and shoot directly into the most primitive part of our brain, the limbic system. Here sits the emotional brain and the core of the autonomic nervous system. The nose is a portal to the brain, and the brain is raw to the world through the nose.

The aroma's imprint on the brain causes old memories, thoughts, and emotions to resurface, or creates new ones on the first whiff, whether we want it to or not. The new emotional response simultaneously creates corresponding biochemical messengers, known as neuropeptides. These chemical messengers are sent to receptor cites on cell membranes throughout the body. They tell the cell how to behave. Cells create tissue.

"Neuropeptides and their receptors are the biochemicals of emotion. The emotions are the informational content that is exchanged via the psychosomatic network, with the many systems, organs, and cells participating in the process. Like information, then, the emotions travel between the two realms of mind and body, as the peptides and their receptors in the physical realm, and as the feelings we experience and call emotions in the nonmaterial realm… by definition, information belongs to neither mind nor body, although it touches both."
Candace B. Pert, PhD, *Molecules of Emotion*

Simply by inhaling a certain aroma, we can shift from stressful emotions and tight tissue to relief in both realms. Emotional release can be a whiff away, and then the body shifts according to the instructions from the new chemical messengers circulating the body. Happy thoughts create happy cells. *Your* Inner River of Peace is sustained. Oh, how important it is to honor and control our thoughts and feelings. They create our words and actions and our future self.

The response to an aroma could be peaceful or it could be stressful. It could be joyful or full of frustration. Aromas demand we honor the individuality of each of us. This part of their true beauty is serving us to be more and more of our best Self.

In the 1990s when people walked into my Oil Lady Aromatherapy® shop in Naples, Florida, if they were breathing, they got aromatic molecules traveling up their nose. Some got tears in their eyes just from stepping through the door. Often this brought up memories of their homeland, grandmothers, or a way of life that honored essential oils and aromas. Sometimes it simply awakened a yearning in their hearts for compassion. The comment we often heard: *Umm, this feels like home.*

The electromagnetic frequency of essential oils is a fully recognized reality measurable by science. Many frequencies of essential oils go beyond the measurable frequency of a healthy body and the healthiest of foods and herbs.

Essential oils are drops of liquid for the health of our physical body and drops of light for our nonphysical mind, emotions, and spirit. These qualities enable them to deliver their medicine and message to the different levels and dimensions of our being. It happens simultaneously with wonder and awe. It still makes me go silent, makes my heart smile, and takes me to my knees when I observe this happening in others.

Essential oils, with their medicine and message, offer extraordinary support for our whole self. Our physical, mental, and spiritual worlds are all embraced as one. There are no lines of differentiation. We are supported, sustained and regenerated with essential oils playing their role as a big aromatic holy comforter. Essential oils occupy a huge platter on the buffet table of healing games and good medicine.

Essential oils, as microcosms of holistic medicine, are functioning examples of epigenetics.

This brief and over simplified explanation of epigenetics is included here to show the integral part essential oils play in our health on all levels. The epigenetic chain of events is one of the reasons the soulful elements of essential oils fulfill their mission.

Epigenetics is a new field of biology. Science previously recognized the nucleus of the cell as the cell's brain, controlling the development of our genes. Epigenetics is the discovery that protein receptors on cell membranes receive the neuropeptide information and pass it into the cells. The cells behavior is based on this information which effects the activity of our genes. Thus, the cell membrane is now considered to be the cell's brain, not the nucleus. Any biochemical information of any kind that attaches to the receptor sites on cell membranes has a direct effect on the cell's behavior including our genes.

Essential oils work through the skin since they are lipid soluble. Thus, they have direct access into the blood stream. Through the nose, they have direct access to the brain and lungs. The chemical messengers that are created from these effects are sent to cell membrane receptor sites through our body. As the cellular activity changes, so goes the tissue.

Essential oils can be seen as a form of nutrition for our body, mind, soul, and spirit. With their liquid and aroma, they are a silent conscious and unconscious language. This provides an environment and a terrain enveloping our whole self, and the environment in which we live. When we are inhaling an essential oil, the aroma effects those around us. Aromatic molecules live and travel in the air we all breathe together.

Thus, essential oils are truly an element of integrative, complementary and functional medicine. Essential oils are a living example of the interconnectedness of the whole being. They do not treat us as a bundle of separate parts. Original medicine of indigenous peoples had medicine women and men that *saw* our wholeness. Modern medicine started dividing up our parts to be treated separately. Now we are returning to the wisdom, compassion and power of holistic medicine.

Essential oils on their Royal Mission are bringing our scattered parts back together. All the while they are building up our compassion for ourselves, others, and nature. Their liquid and aroma are portals into our Inner River of Peace. The historical, present, and future story of essential oils is exciting and inspirational.

The Royal Mission of Essential Oils

With the strength of an equilateral triangle, we see the Royal Mission of essential oils in the power of threes.

Due to their natural chemical constituents and exquisite aromas, these precious liquids provided by Mother Nature serve us exquisitely well. They also serve the plant and animal kingdoms. We were all created to have a symbiotic relationship anchored in deep respect and compassion. This is crucial to our survival and our ability to joyfully thrive with a renewed abundance mentality.

The vision-intention-purpose for this book is to build the connection with *your* Inner River of Peace. When we meet with this vision, the relationship strengthens. Using The Messages with essential oils is one of the best examples of how their Royal Mission is assimilated as a form of nourishment. My personal and professional relationship with essential oils has taught me the vast scope of influence essential oils have on our health and our life. They have an innate ability to reveal certain parts of ourselves that need want attention, while assisting us in following our dreams with courage and compassion.

First and foremost, essentials oils are here to guide us into our Inner River of Peace while we travel the *Path of Our Personal Legend* (Paulo Coelho). Essential oils give us magnificent ways to create and enjoy all kinds of *holy habits*. Continually getting our true self in order is a soul call unique to each of us. It is also a continual lifetime expedition of compassion and purpose. We find opportunities to get better and better every day. What we are is what we give to the world.

Essential oils first meet us on a personal level, honoring wherever we are. Thus, they:

1. **Assist** us through life transitions of all kinds, including getting up in the morning and going to bed at night, changing jobs and homes, handling relationship changes, being born and passing away.
2. **Protect** our health on the physical, mental, and spiritual planes, including illnesses and soul calls.
3. **Celebrate** each day and event of our lives and remind us to celebrate our whole self, including

the clarity and courage to step through the next open door.

They have a three-step purpose for each of us which empowers our relationship with our Inner River of Peace. Thus, they:

1. **Bring our scattered parts back together**. The physical and nonphysical properties of essential oils bring our physical form and nonphysical realm into harmony. Acquiring healthy self-love is the question, the answer, the lock, and the key.

2. Once we start to bring our own parts into balance, we are able to meet others here and start to **understand the true oneness of us all.** Compassion for others is an extension of the love we have for our self.

3. Then on a third level, with love and compassion in our hearts powered by our Inner River of Peace, we are able to **restore our reverent connection with nature**. We are regenerated from this relationship and can then remember to honor life in all things great and small.

Essential oils come into our lives for a reason, a season, or a lifetime. Our love for certain essential oils can change just as we change. Our body serves as a temple for the soul and a vessel for our spirit. It also is a chemistry tube constantly popping and fizzling to maintain homeostasis as we pass through the seasons of life. The space suit we are in requires constant supervision and continual maintenance. This is part of the human dilemma.

Thus, essential oils are here for a:

1. **Reason** - to soothe, such as a headache, aching muscles, a cold, cut, or a burn.
2. **Season** - to smooth the transitions in life and take off the rough edges or to celebrate the shift, such as with menopause, relocations, new jobs, new relationships, losses of loved ones, and illnesses.
3. **Lifetime** - to provide a soul affinity with a certain aroma. This aroma melts your heart into a place of grace. This stillness holds a sense of being home in yourself. The aromatic imprint is the key of you on the musical scale of smell. I call this our personal harmonic convergence of the sympathetic and parasympathetic sides of the autonomic nervous system. How lovely.

Example: One of my soul affinities is with the aroma of Rose otto (*Rosa damascena*) pure essential oil of Bulgaria. This was realized

Essential Oils as Soulful Elements

in England when studying with the late Madame Micheline Arcier of London. I was her seventh and last student in the United States. This was the first time I smelled genuine Rose otto. My thought was: *Wow, now **this** is the real smell of rose.* It felt like my whole being was melting down with a silky diamond liquid plasma. This beautiful vapor of love appeared just by breathing. With the first whiff, I was home. Some part of me just *knew* rose. A window of knowledge, wisdom, and love opened up. This Inner River of Peace experience was of the highest order.

Rose is sent to the earth by the gardeners of paradise for empowering the mind and the eye of the spirit.
Rumi

This is true only if you love the aroma of roses. Any genuine aroma of essential oils can make you feel this way for a reason, a season, or a lifetime. Find the essential oils that are yours to love. Their love for you is boundaryless.

Essential oils deliver special wisdom unique to each of us in a timely way. They walk their talk. They get our immediate attention by zapping us into the present moment, or if necessary, they will zap us out of the present moment with much needed relief. They offer many kinds of wisdom.

1. **Less is often more.** Too much of an essential oil for too long can give us a worse headache than the one we are trying to relieve. Too much lavender or tea tree on troubled skin spots reaches a tipping point for healing, and the spot gets red and irritated again.

2. **Just enough is just enough.** The right essential oil, in right dosage and method of delivery, for the right length of time is just enough.

3. Their aroma demands we **honor the individuality** in each of us. This is due to our life experiences and memories, personal constitution, and our primitive emotional and unconscious brain.

As our parts and systems come back into homeostasis, our physical and nonphysical parts start to dance and flow in harmony. Our mental, emotional, and spiritual worlds start to come together. We can connect to our Inner River of Peace on a grand scale. Simply put, we feel a lot better. We think, feel, speak, and act differently. Our brain releases biochemistry based on the new thoughts and emotions. Our heart-mind muscle lights up like a golden nugget and a diamond. We are in the smooth clear waters of our Inner River of Peace.

Essential Oils as Soulful Elements

Essential oils are compassionate companions with The Messages in delivering their wisdom and love. Strengthening this connection with *your* Inner River of Peace is the dream-goal. Essential oils with their physical highly concentrated volatile liquids and their nonphysical intense vaporous aromas, provide a powerful multi-level soulful element to anchor us in this river. We find a soothing and comforting experience amidst the dross of life.

The role of essential oils for us is the same for plant life. They serve life on the planet, drop by drop, molecule by molecule, one creature and one plant at a time. Their purpose is to:

1. **Assist** the plant world with growth and reproduction.
2. **Protect** plants from disease and predators. The aroma attracts lovers and repels predators.
3. **Celebrate** the flowers and the fruits as they bloom and live out their purpose.

Even if we use essential oils only for inhalation, they will be *working* their Royal Mission with The Messages. They will also be soothing your troubled mind, calming your emotions, and supporting your immune system. Then they will be celebrating all that you are as you continue to *Show Up and Hold the Vision* (Message One) of the power in *your* Inner River of Peace. You also might find yourself sleeping better. Essential oils have their physical properties, and then they have their vaporous invisible aromas with their beautiful and mysterious ways. As masters, they meet us right where we are and show us the way forward. How lovely.

Focus on the Light and Love
and That is what You will magnify.

Message Three

What a beautiful thing it is to focus light and love on The Messages enhanced with sacred oils and their aromas. *Holy habits create holy happenings.* Tremendous blessings and gratitude are found here.

Note: Anosmia is the loss of our sense of smell. Your sense of smell may be gone due to one of many reasons or it may be very weak. Sometimes it can get better; sometimes it can come back. It may well be worth exploring. From experience, I recommend inhaling pure straight peppermint essential oil from a small bottle. People have reported they can feel the tingling sensation in their nose from the menthol stimulation even when they can't smell the aroma. Let this stimulation of the olfactory neurons do their work. Notice any changes in how you might feel.

Ten Essential Oils

Here we review ten of the essential oils mentioned throughout the Ten Messages. The purpose of using essential oils with The Messages is to experience the sacred synergy between them. This is a quick and powerful way to anchor deeply in *your* Inner River of Peace.

Therefore, with this purpose in our heart-mind muscle, be sure you really love the way the aroma makes you feel. All you need to do is inhale the pure essential oil while repeating The Message. Your heart opens and calls in your spirit. Enjoy your renewed sense of well-being.

> *Look into the perfumes of flowers and of nature*
> *for peace of mind and joy of life.*
> Wang Wei

Consider using essential oils with The Messages as elements of liquid peace. They offer aromatic comfort while delivering the wisdom and love from each Message. Along with this, comes the joy of being on our path of perfect fulfillment. We are being regenerated for that of which we were created. This is available in the unlimited field of possibilities that lives in the power that goes way beyond.

The following are some of the characteristics suggesting why these essential oils might serve among your choices to accompany The Messages. Instead of thinking it out, let your nose guide you. The nose knows what we need and bypasses the thinking mind. Each essential oil below is matched with a Message only to give examples of one way to use them. Match them up as you wish.

Lavender (*Lavandula augustifolia*) is the # 1 Balancer of essential oils for the central nervous system. Lavender is from the Latin word *lavare* meaning to wash and clear. This is true for the mental-focused head as well as the whole body. Its gentle smooth aroma embodies peace and calmness. The colors of lavender flowers with green leaves unite the mind and heart. It is the most desirable essential oil for the most people to relieve stress.

> *What are you fretting about? Don't you remember?*
> *All YOU agreed to do is:*
> *Show Up and Hold the Vision.*
> *We can do all the rest through you.*   *Message One*

Orange (*Citrus sinensis*) has a sweet and nurturing aroma. Orange tends to make people smile, bring up yummy memories, and shift heavy anxious feelings. It carries the sparkling energy of the sun and the joyfulness of a child. As a sweet fruit of life, it offers a comforting respite to our scattered parts. The nurturing embrace of orange reveals the sweetness of possibilities.

> *Whenever you Think you are limited,*
> *Look at the Sky.*   *Message Two*

Peppermint (*Mentha piperita*) is warming and cooling, uplifting and calming. It knows which one we need. The zap of menthol cuts to the quick and sharpens our mental focus. Peppermint clears the head and the lungs, and aids digestion. We see clearly, breathe with ease, and digest our thoughts and feelings with uplifting insights. With increased awareness and new perceptions, we receive the wisdom from The Messages.

> *Focus on the Light and Love*
> *and That is what You will magnify.*   Message Three

Sandalwood (*Santalum album*) inspires the deep rich stillness of prayer and meditation. The cooling and soothing qualities have a sedative effect in the nervous system. As an oil of antiquity, sandalwood is valued and honored for its deep tranquility and divine wisdom. The rich viscous essential oil anchors us in the body, while its silky-smooth aroma touches the soul. With the ability to unite the heaven and earth within us, it taps into the universal truth of The Messages, with devotion to The Messenger.

> *Anchor way down deep*
> *in the bottom of the ocean,*
> *and ride the waves.*
> *Everything is OK.*   Message Four

Eucalyptus (*Eucalyptus radiata*) is stimulating and revitalizing as a top oil of respiration. The fresh crisp aroma enhances our breathing and opens the chest area. Eucalyptus provides the opportunity to experience freedom from past blocks or stagnation. Inspiration with respiration is a form of renewal. From inhalation, the reflex reaction creates deep breathing for the brain and the lungs.

It moves the rivers in the body. This centering and openness allow us to awaken and breathe in our dreams, our spirit, and our Inner River of Peace. The Messenger reminds us of our role.

> *Keep Me with you,*
> *just Keep Me with you.*   *Message Five*

Geranium (*Pelargonium roseum*) is a silky-smooth restful yin oil for balancing the feminine energies in all of us. With calm strength, it nourishes the feminine creative and life-giving ways of the thinking heart and the feeling mind that unite with the sacral center. As a nurturing aromatic comforter, geranium (with its rose qualities) releases frazzled nerves and overwhelming thoughts and emotions. Our imagination and intuition are awakened with new thoughts and insights. We receive messages of love, reminding us to release resistance and frustration.

> *Don't resist, pull, push, or struggle*
> *in the web of this life you're in.*
> *Everyone is in the web of life.*
> *Be there with it, in all its turmoil, and peace shall prevail.*
>   *Message Six*

Frankincense (*Boswellia carterii*) is the protector with its strength and power. As an oil of antiquity, frankincense serves to enhance our spiritual and mental sense of well-being, as it protects the health of our body. Deepening our breath, it restores the flow of life force energy by settling the mind and soothing the emotions. Like sandalwood, frankincense serves us humans well as a reverent essential oil for quiet contemplation, carrying the wisdom and love from The Messages.

> *The Power out here is much great than anything you can ever imagine, even when you Think you are in your most expanded state.*
> *It goes way beyond that.* — Message Seven

Neroli (*Citrus aurantium v. amara*) ushers in a breath of heaven from the flowers at the top of the orange trees. The high-pitched delicate aroma lifts us above the dross of life. As a precious and dear essential oil of the highest vibrations, it offers radiant light to release old patterns and instill a purity of spirit. It lifts us up to the light-infused colors of the *Love Rainbow of Trust,* where we are also asked to trust our whole self. Soothing anxious and fearful worries of the heart, it reveals love and peace as The Messages offer their insights and wisdom. Embrace The Messenger's invitation.

> *You must Trust me like never before, if you want to survive.* — Message Eight

Helichrysum (*Helichrysum italicum or augustifolia*), also known as Immortelle and Everlasting, serves us well with exceptional healing properties for stagnant physical and emotional challenges. The smooth flowing liquid bathes wounded tissue and a fearful mind. Like clear spring water, it moves the rivers, while calmly and patiently guiding us through the healing process. With inspiration to embrace the pain, it soothes the heart and comforts our soul. Forgiveness and wisdom from The Messages soothe the transformation from stagnation to liberation and compassion. This inner strength taps into the healing and accepting love in The Messages.

> *The Coal of your life has made you
> into The Diamond that you are.*   *Message Nine*

Rose otto (*Rosa damascena*) is the Oil of the Heart and Queen of the Flowers. Rose is a universal and historical symbol of divine love. This dear essential oil has a regulating effect on our whole system and nourishes the heart, while restoring a sense of well-being. This clear liquid light with an exceptionally high frequency is an offering of pure floral aroma to clear heat and inflammation physically, emotionally and spiritually. She shows us the genuine power of gentle. Easing sorrows with a loving soothing embrace, rose serves as a Holy Comforter and a symbol of God's love for the world. It envelops each Message with the love of The Messenger.

> *You are Called where you are called
> to experience my Love.*   *Message Ten*

Essential Oils as Soulful Elements

Essential oils hold the wisdom of the ages, as Mother Nature offers us her most precious liquid from her plants and trees. Their natural medicinal properties such as antibacterial, antiviral, and anti-inflammatory provide protection and healing for our bodies. The aroma from these highly concentrated volatile liquids, assists us in releasing, restoring and regenerating our mental, emotional, and spiritual worlds that are too often depleted. Our heart-mind muscle thrives as our spirit and soul soar.

Ideas for the aromas you love:
1. Use the same essential oil for all The Messages.
2. Use a different one for each Message.
3. Use a combination of essential oils for the first nine Messages, and a separate one for Message Ten.

What to do:

Most of all be creative and invent your very own heart-warming and mind-soothing *holy habits* that speak to your soul through essentials oils and their companion Messages. Dream, explore, and discover. Do and be this for your holy self. Remember how precious you really are.

Remember to be *Slow, Still, and Simple (SSS)*. Essential oils show us there is power in simple.

For the purpose of enhancing each Message using the sense of smell with genuine essential oils, here are some simple and highly effective methods of use to consider. Experiment and see if one or two are just right for you. Keep your heart-mind muscle on The Message as you breathe in the vaporous aromas of peace.

1. **Inhale** a pure straight genuine essential oil from a small bottle or on a cotton ball and keep it with you. Use the Simple Focused-Breathing Technique at the end of each Message. Inhalation alone is enough to get it all. It's just enough.

2. **Mist** with one drop of essential oil per two ounces of good water. Shake well before each misting. *Touch With Oils® Misting Technique:*
   - Circle the top of your head at arm's length. Circle in the direction your arm and hand go naturally. There is no right or wrong way.
   - Next, come down and mist your face.
   - Then, closely mist the back of your neck in the center, just below the hair line with three close zaps right on the skin.

Essential Oils as Soulful Elements

- Close your eyes with The Message and breathe slowly.

3. **Make a palm blend** by adding one drop of essential oil in 1-2 pumps of a base oil, lotion or cream in your palm. Rub your palms together spreading the blend out to your fingertips. You tap into your heart through the palms of your hands. Feel the blessing of what you are doing. Give thanks for this oil of gladness. Now you are ready to enjoy your palm blend. You can do one or more of the following:

Touch With Oils® Anointing Technique:

- First, apply some of the blend to the outside of your nostrils (to make the nose-brain connection).
- Second, gently place the pads of your fingers on your temples making gentle slow circles with your fingers *attached* to the skin (not moving over the skin).
- Third, move to the back of your neck below the hairline making the same gentle slow circles.
- Fourth, make small gentle circles on your heart area.

- Lastly, rub your palms together again, and cup your hands over your nose. Close your eyes and breathe slowly. Pause and be still while repeating your Message. Be full-of-thanks for this comforting way to nurture the wholeness of yourself.

Try doing steps 2 through 4 right now with slow circles using the soft pads of your fingers. Notice a little shift that happens with your breathing and how you feel.

Use the above technique as a prayer when awakening to the new day with a stimulating essential oil in a palm blend, or to tuck yourself in at night for sweet sleep with a calming palm blend. You can also visualize the technique at any time. The mind doesn't know the difference between what is real and what is visualized/imagined. The body responds accordingly to the *molecules of emotion* created in the brain.

Any of the five steps, even one or two, can be done by themselves. Try this as a *holy habit* in a lovely bath or a great shower.

Essential Oils as Soulful Elements

Let your nose guide you with each essential oil and each Message.

See how they resonate together. For example, if we are overwhelmed and stressed while we are trying to develop our skill to *Show Up and Hold the Vision*, then lavender might really deliver the goods since it is the #1 balancer for our whole nervous system. This is true if we love the aroma. Delight in the exploration of this process. It is fun to learn how different aromas affect us. There are things to uncover here.

Once you use a certain aroma with a Message, keep them together to reinforce their imprint on the brain and the heart. The aroma and The Message create a nose-brain entrainment. This occurs simply by inhaling the aroma while repeating The Message. Together they share the same mental and emotional response. When you smell the aroma, or repeat The Message, one brings up the memory of the other. The body relaxes accordingly. The Inner River of Peace comes forth.

Precautions with Essential Oils

Keep safety in mind always. Since essential oils are pure and natural, the tendency is if some is good, then more is better. Wisdom in using essential oils reveals less is often more.

Once the right essential oil and dosage is formulated, using too much for too long goes past the tipping point of healing. It can irritate the skin, create an extreme sensitivity and become toxic to the entire system. It can also have adverse effects with certain medications.

All substances are poisonous;
there is none that is not a poison.
The right dose differentiates a poison from a remedy.
Paracelsus, 16th Century Alchemist

Lavender was my first love in the essential oil world. It was in the first aromatherapy massage that relieved my physical pain, mental stress and emotional exhaustion all at once. There were times in massage and in baths I was out of pain with lavender. Geranium was the other essential oil that added to this blessing.

After years of pouring and using essential oils in my professional practice, I developed such a sensitivity to lavender that I could no longer use it. This can happen with any and all essential oils. Time has proven this to be true for many of us with decades in the industry. This is not unusual with extreme exposure. Too much of the most wonderful things, like water and essential oils, can pass the peak of good health.

Essential oils are highly concentrated volatile liquids. They do not mix with water. They are lipid (fat) soluble. This means they are excellent for mixing in bases of oils, creams, and lotions, as well as milk and cream.

Apart from spot work, such as one drop of lavender on a burn of unbroken skin, or a drop as perfume, they are too strong to use consistently undiluted on the skin. Many essential oils can cause skin irritations. Once they are on the skin, since they are lipid soluble, they are in the body. Even with blends, it is wise to do a skin test first with a dab of the blend.

Essential oils are too strong for internal use without professional medical advice. They can burn internal tissue in the mouth, throat, and intestines. Many hospital visits have resulted from internal use or straight use on the skin. One person burned their throat swallowing essential oil in some water and ended up in the hospital on a feeding tube. Another person put straight oregano on a baby's arm. This burn put the baby in the hospital.

In general, the rules are:

- Keep essential oils away from children, pets, and open flames.
- Children, pregnant mothers, and sensitive situations require professional advice.
- All essential oils are not safe for aromatherapy use. Some can be toxic or be contraindicated with some medications.

- Others can create undesirable effects depending on the person, their age, and their condition.
- Take care of yourself and loved ones with good education and professional advice.

Respect and reverence for essential oils and nature is reflected in the quality of our survival. The earth is our only supplier, and some essential oils are diluted and adulterated to meet the market demands. Preserving nature as our source for food, shelter, medicine, enrichment, and spiritual evolution is our human responsibility. Conscientious use benefits everyone.

With more people on the planet than ever before, the population demands more natural resources. Some of the root causes of these challenges include:

1. Loss of our Inner River of Peace in a chaotic, complicated, confused, and changing world.
2. Loss of our connection to community and loss of our compassion for others.
3. Loss of our connection to nature which challenges the well-being and existence of the earth, animals, and humans.

The Messages keep us on track as we *Show Up and Hold the Vision* and *Focus on the Light and Love*. The connection to *your* Inner River of Peace is a bond to be cherished, honored, nurtured, and held in a special place in your heart. The Messages show us the way, and essential oils show up to assist them. Be full of gratitude every chance you can.

Review

If you decide to use essential oils with your Messages, the most important issue is to choose the ones that really speak to your heart. The more you like the aroma, the quicker and deeper the results. An aroma we love makes us automatically breathe deeper and pause. We feel good. It's an aromatic autonomic reflex response. This requires no thinking or struggling to make something happen.

Essential oils are *stars of medicine* and lights of divinity. The silent power of aroma with the silent power of The Message, ushers in the silent wisdom and love from The Messenger. A soulful return to our Inner River of Peace can last for minutes or days. Be gracious for this. Life is precious, and so are you.

Silence is the element in which great things fashion themselves.
Thomas Carlyle

Essential oils are a language of no words. The silent aroma brings us into the present moment and helps us find our way forward, all in the name of love. The experiences I shared with people from other cultures, whose languages I couldn't speak, would have been diminished with words. The connecting conduit is the Inner River of Peace. Essential oils are liquid aromatic drops from this River of Peace that flows through all of us and is deeply *seeded* within. They can dissolve the barriers between people and cultures.

Essential oils are fashioned to exquisitely help us find our life's course. They have the amazing glorious ability to calm the scattered mind, open our heart, and call in our spirt. Their timing in life is of the Divine. In a loving way, they give us the courage to follow the guidance. With this comes a faith and trust that keeps getting stronger, as does our relationship with our Inner River of Peace.

The body affects the mind and the mind affects the body. Essential oils swirl them together like a figure-eight. They are integrally integrated through nature's magnificent design. Our soul and spirit calmly and silently rejoice when this happens. The field of possibility awaits.

All this can happen when we use essential oils as soulful elements to bring our scattered parts back together with the wisdom and love from The Messages.

1. One drop
2. One breath
3. One touch (physical or nonphysical) at a time.

Make a conscious effort to slow down with your *holy habits*, be still for a few breaths, and realize how simple techniques add

Essential Oils as Soulful Elements

richness to your life. They go with you wherever you are, and enable you to travel lightly. Oh, the places you can go from here.

As you *Show Up and Hold the Vision*, remember to hold your *Focus on the Light and Love.* The power available goes beyond our grandest imagination.

Essential oils are Soulful Elements with a Royal Mission for humans. They bring our scattered yet holy parts together, bring us all together through the Inner River of Peace, and reunite us with the earth. They naturally assist us through our transitions, protect our health on all levels, and remind us to celebrate more and more of our whole self.

Aroma is the silent language of the soul.

Build Your Own Home of Cards

The more ways we have to welcome The Messages in our lives, the more of their wisdom and love comes in for us. The power of repetition in developing muscles and creating new habits is well known to all of us. The Ten Messages of Love give us the opportunity to strengthen our creative abilities, to trust our intuition, and to explore our imagination. The repetition of all these gifts brings us home to our Inner River of Peace.

I love to write. Since high school, I've kept journals and lists of favorite quotes. I have index cards of Messages and passages that really speak to me. They are continual reminders of the strong, loving relationship I am choosing to keep building with my whole self. I still cherish these cards as *holy habits* that are meaningful to me. They are very much alive and abide in a special place in my heart and mind. They strengthen and support my heart-mind muscle, which is always an ongoing adventure. On either my bedside table or on my morning desk, my cards have a spot in my line of sight. Some are rather ear-torn and faded. A few became many, and then many became more over the years.

There are about thirty or so that are my core cards I keep active. Others are kept in my desk to draw upon as desired. Sometimes, I'll shuffle this deck and pull out one or two cards. It's just right for what I needed. The cards help keep my perspective open to receive any new ways to see and think. They remind me what I want to keep cultivating, as well as what I love about myself and don't want to lose. Through the years, I continue to read them in the morning and/or night. The words continue to mean more to me as I gain more life experiences. The Messages stay the same (because they are not my words); the other cards often get tweaked and updated.

At least once a year, I like to review the cards and make some changes or additions for where life has taken me at that time. It's a space and time for revision and renewal with these inspiring words and feelings. For many years, I have been taking a week off in the beginning of January to disengage from life the best I can. My husband and I do this together now. Nature plays a big role in where we go. Often, it's the beach, the mountains, a prayer house, or another place of soulful elements. One time it was an inn in Santa Fe, another it was the Everglades Lodge in Everglades City, Florida. Each year shows us the place.

The beginning of January is quiet almost everywhere, and even with business most people don't really need you that week. This provides a stillness in time and a sacred space to stop the busyness of life, look over the past year, and listen to what the next year wants to be. Then we come down off the mountain and back into the village to embark on the coming year in a conscious way. My core cards are with me, and some new ones or adjusted ones are added to my mission for the year. This is a contemplative time to anchor our strength in our relationship with the higher power of The Messenger. The dream-goal is to start off the year with our Inner River of Peace with us.

Times for reflection, review, and renewal are part of the healing games and good medicine one must play, just to remain sane. Our ability to imagine, be inspired, and connect to our intuition, leads us to the everlasting and continually evolving invention of who we are. This leads to the further discovery of what we are here to do and be. Sometimes it is simply being the goodness of who we are. This is enough.

Explore the idea of having The Messenger's Ten Messages of Love on "cards." Honor each message with its own card. This leaves room for a date or a note over the days, weeks, and maybe even years as The Messages are reflected upon in different life events. Most of my cards have dates with a word or two scribbled in some corner or place on the card.

The value of a card is the ability to touch it, take it with you, see The Message easily, and add a note through the action of writing. The hand is an outward expression of the inward heart. Touching or reading the card or writing a word or two, means we have paused. Our focus and breath have shifted for a few moments. Our very own home of cards can turn into *holy habits* and inspire us to *Stop, Look and Listen (SLL)* and be *Slow, Still and Simple (SSS)*. Here we find an increased peace of mind.

Maybe you are not a writer or card person. The field of infinite possibilities is open to you. Let your imagination bring you some wonderful ideas. Invent your own way to honor The Messages as they honor you. Discover a way to keep them in your life. At different times in our lives, they keep showing up as wisdom teachers and take us deeper into our Inner River of Peace. This means we are exploring more and more about ourselves and gaining some new

Build Your Own Home of Cards

perspectives. The more we do this, the more we find our heart-mind muscle at work (love made visible). Giving and receiving become one when we are connected to our Inner River of Peace.

There are many advantages to having each Message on a card, such as an index card or something smaller. You can take one with you wherever you go, put one on the mirror, or put it in a special holder on your desk or eating table. Shuffle the deck and pull a card for that moment, day, or event. Let it work for you and serve you well.

Each time I take a trip, I see the adventure as a kind of pilgrimage. Trips and travels are good times to focus on a Message you want to keep with you. Be open to what is waiting for you. At the end of a trip, I ask myself: *What was the pearl, golden nugget, or diamond I went on the trip to find?* It provides a few contemplative moments of reflection. There is always wisdom waiting to be invited in and found.

Maybe you like to draw, color or paint. Over the years I have written The Messages on greeting cards that I still paint in watercolor. I love sending them to friends, and their responses are so genuinely grateful. Some tell me they keep them on the refrigerator or bathroom mirror. What joy this is to have a reminder right in front of your face. Eye level is hard to miss.

Discover your *holy habits* to keep The Messages in your life.
Build your own home of cards to serve you well.
It is yours to create.

Living with The Messenger and The Messages is something to be cherished. There are times we wonder where they are, and other times they are a tower of strength. Having them on cards or in a journal, helps us keep going in the daily-doings amidst the dross in the world. There is beauty to be found. As we gain the insights, wisdom and love, we start realizing how courageous and wonderful we are. Our desire to deeply keep moving forward, while courageously standing tall, is why we are here.

These ten Messages were not ever just for me. Now they are here for you, and perhaps some others you know. *The Circle of Compassion in Action* is available to all in search of their Inner River of Peace. As long as there is still one pearl, one diamond, or one golden nugget to be found, the dream-goal for this book is at work as *love made visible*. One by one, drop by drop, the Inner River of Peace lights up one person at a time.

Remember The Messenger's words in Message Ten.

*You are Called where you are called
to experience my Love.*

May the Ten Messages of Love show you *your* Inner River of Peace. Here you are nourished, nurtured, and blessed with the compassionate waters of peace offering glimpses of infinite love.

What Happened Here?

I am here at the end of my book-story, thanking you for your willingness to *Show Up and Hold the Vision* of *your* Inner River of Peace. Writing my stories that called in The Messenger with these Ten Messages of Love, presented endless possibilities for ways to come home to the marriage of my heart and mind over and over again.

The reason I dug deeper into all these Messages with these writings is because I believe I was writing for others who will experience a new enlightened sense of well-being. The Messages are a gift with no expiration date and continue to teach me how they can be applied to just about everything. Regardless of age, condition, or culture, life is better with The Messenger offering us Ten Messages of Love.

So, what happened for me? To write my book, meant I was called to live deeper with each Message along with each of my personal stories. I lived with some Messages for several weeks; others took longer to write. Reliving each life event from the perspective of where I am now in life, continued to reveal more golden nuggets. I honor and cherish The Messages even more than the first time I heard them. Then there were more revisits with each edit. There appeared to be another level of brilliance added to the diamonds. This has continued to be a lifetime adventuresome challenge of worthy ideals.

I also lived with the four *Message Reviews* consisting of several messages together, and I encourage you to do the same. I saw The Messages as best friends who make each other better just by being together. This was a new realization for me and was not part of the original vision for the book. Supporting each other, The Messages create a continuum of spirit, wisdom, and love that travels on the *Love Rainbow of Trust*.

The farther along I got in the book the more I saw the Inner River of Peace flowing through the book and connecting The Messages. With this sacred synergy, I noticed as I was writing about

What Happened Here?

one Message, one of the others would come in with a word or two to contribute. They kept popping in with my heart-mind muscle to flow through the book with the other Messages. They serve each other, just like we are meant to serve each other. They do not thrive as well on their own, as they do together. There is much wisdom here. It called me to *Stop, Look and Listen (SLL)*.

The meaning, wisdom and love being offered with each Message, goes beyond anything I imagined. Again, throughout my life, they continue to help me discover and live my personal mission as it grows, changes and winds around each bend. I love seeing this evolution with childlike eyes-of-wonder. The unknowns in our life will eventually become known out of the powerful field that has no limits. The Messages teach me to embrace and trust the unknowns the best I can. They continue to show me miracles, mystery and eventually grace.

The Messages became stronger as they were written through my heart and hands again. They provided clarity in their purpose and in my purpose on an expansive level. They reminded me of my dreams and continued to give me inspiration and courage to keep writing. The dreams in my waking and sleep states have been enriched through this writing experience.

It takes courage and trust to live these lives on a daily basis. Often, I wondered how in the world it was going to be possible to get this book of love written and published. So, I looked at the dream-goal with my heart, and then put my head down and kept writing—page by page, chapter by chapter. In the last year of writing, I spent four different weeks at the beach, a week at the monastery, many days in the library, early mornings in my studio, and afternoons at the dining room table or in my yellow room. Then I would think of Aristotle and go for a walk to *Stop, Look, and Listen (SLL)*. The answer was always: honor the value of *Slow, Still, and Simple (SSS)*. Sometimes, I would go slow, just as fast as I could. When I felt overwhelmed, Message One kept showing up to remind me I was simply the vessel.

> *What are you fretting about? Don't you remember?*
> *All YOU agreed to do is:*
> *Show Up and Hold the Vision.*
> *We can do all the rest through you.*

The Messages continued to guide me as I wrote the book. They became a highly effective performance team as their momentum continued to build from Message One through Message Ten. They know the truth of the ways of existence. With God, as The Messenger, the wisdom and love from each Message prevailed though each section of the book. When I got tired or blocked, I practiced one or more of my *holy habits*.

What Happened Here?

The writing experience called me to live each Message and reminded me of my childlike sense of wonder that loves my Inner River of Peace. Who were your favorite characters? Peter Pan, Tinkerbell, Alice in Wonderland, Pocahontas, and Annie Oakley are a few of mine. Don't let the ways of the world take the energy and memories of those characters away from you. The Messages hold delightful secrets of all kinds.

How about you? Do you have some new perceptions with some new meaningful *holy habits* to accompany The Messenger and The Messages? Are you realizing *your* Inner River of Peace is here for you? If you are standing on the riverbank, jump or ease yourself into the river with The Messages and your *holy habits* in your chest pocket near your heart. Ask and pray with all your heart and mind for what you need to know every time you want it. Be aware, the answer comes in many forms, many places and many different times.

- **Invite** The Message in by **asking** The Messenger for the loving guidance.
- **Embrace** it with all your heart and mind.
- **Be full** of thanksgiving ahead of time for what you **trust** will appear.

We're all searching for our Inner River of Peace the best we can. You are a radiant drop of water, vibrating out into rippling rings that touch the people around you. This happens just by *being* who you are.

I can only imagine the wonderful things God has instore for you. The Messenger is here to guide us and love us with the amazingly glorious Great Holy Comforter of Light and Love. All of us and all of the world are yearning for this now more than ever. The adventuresome challenges come and go. The Inner River of Peace prevails.

I send you the *Love Rainbow of Trust* that is blessed
by the Grace of God.

Conclusion

I believe the dream-goal of my book-story is living in some part of you, as you have **Shown Up and Held the Vision** for *your* Inner River of Peace.

I believe you have **Looked** at the sky and **Focused** on the light and love, so you are now magnifying your desires and dreams in some way, shape, or form with a sense of adventure.

I believe you have **Anchored** deep and are **Keeping The Messenger** with you in an amazing, sacred, mysterious, and beautiful place in your precious heart and brilliant mind.

I believe you have experienced a sense of **Releasing** some resistance, that *your* Inner River of Peace has prevailed, and there is a knowing that the **Power** from the way beyond is available to assist you.

I believe you are walking on the **Love Rainbow of Trust** and know in every fiber of your being that if you fall off, you can always climb right back on because you *Trust* like never before.

I believe the **Coal** of the tough parts of your past and challenges of the present, are transforming with compassion and grace into the **Diamond** you are today, and that this newfound radiance resonates throughout your whole sense of well-being.

I believe you are enjoying your magnificent and meaningful *holy habits* that remind you of The Messenger, while the wisdom from The Messages keeps you showing up, because you know you are **Called** to experience this omnipresent **Love**.

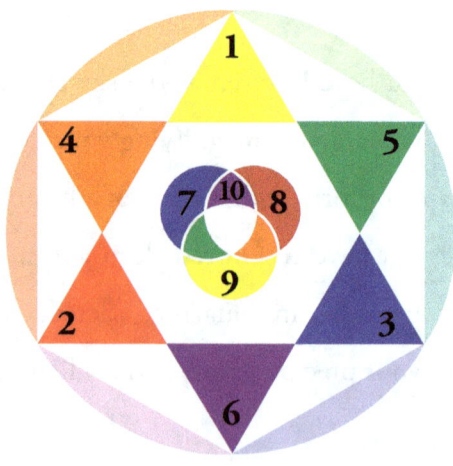

Conclusion

We are all part of this *Circle of Compassion in Action* as it encompasses The Message Mandala and the color wheel of life. Our Inner River of Peace guides us into this field of endless potential and possibilities with the Ten Messages of Love.

My heart's desire is for your realization of the existence and value in developing your heart-mind muscle. Thinking with the heart and feeling with the mind releases the boundaries of their individual realms. There is a renewed sense of wholistic well-being when the heart and mind dance together with The Messages and the power of the senses. Perhaps you have found an essential oil to assist, protect, and celebrate you as the majestic soulful element you are. These are all precious lifetime tools to continue ushering in *your* Inner River of Peace.

Your toolbox of healing games and good medicine is powered by the creation of your own *holy habits* with each Message of Love. In addition, you now have your go-to tools of:

Stop, Look, and Listen (SLL)

Slow, Still, and Simple (SSS)

I encourage you to embrace the adventure of continuing to explore these healing games and good medicine. They are here to guide you through the fast rapids and the stagnant eddies of life. *Your* Inner River of Peace prevails, eventually. Dream and discover how it feels to keep trusting divine timing, divine order, and divine grace every chance you get.

Remember, life is a journey of great courage.

I've always said it takes courage on a daily basis to lead these lives. I keep The Messenger with me the best I know how. After all, what is the alternative?

At age seventy, I have lived with these Messages for years. My life is richer and more blessed because of them. I am still living with them and feel honored to be passing them on to you. Let them continue to serve your yearning heart and scattered mind. Let them guide your way through the ups and downs of life as you trust in the gentle power of the flow.

Most of all, let The Messages inspire you to fully live your once in a lifetime opportunity to be your very best self. When I feel like I've gotten separated from the connection, I hear: *Stay the course; it's still there.*

No matter what happens, don't let go of The Messenger's hand. Remember The Messenger's words:

> *Keep Me with You,*
> *just Keep Me with You*   *Message Five*

> *You are Called where you are called*
> *to experience my Love*   *Message Ten*

Conclusion

Embrace this adventure and see how often The Messages play through you. Drop by drop, embrace each Message as a portal to *your* Inner River of Peace. Each drop effects the river. Therefore, as we bring our scattered parts into harmony, we can then relate to the oneness of the Inner River of Peace in others. From here, we contribute to the ocean of all creation and return to holding a reverence for life with nature and all creatures great and small. It takes many abundant rivers to feed and sustain an ocean.

We can contribute to and become part of the Big Inner River of Peace, Compassion, and Love in the world. The power of this light diminishes the loud rivers of turmoil, chaos, and confusion.

The Messenger and The Messages are here to offer their Royal Service to us humans. There is power, leadership, and a joyful sense of self-worth and belonging that comes to surface from deep within. We each play our own part based on who we truly are.

So, what's next?

I am showing up again and working (as love made visible), on the next set of Ten Messages to further enrich the color wheel of life as a geometric design and Message Mandala, to serve as a compass while traveling *your* Inner River of Peace. God willing and the creek don't rise, Climbing Your Mountain: *One Sacred Step at a Time,* my next book-story, is on its way. I am showing up and focusing light and love on this vision.

Calmness of mind is one of the most beautiful jewels of wisdom.
James Allen

With my heart and mind in sync, I thank you for being here and experiencing a calmness of mind with *your* Inner River of Peace.

In reality you **are** *your* Inner River of Peace.

I believe the Ten Messages of Love have revealed more of *You* to you.

Love is the question, the answer, the lock, and the key.

Life is so very precious—and so are you.

Amen.

Acknowledgements

John Allen Newman, my husband, Knight in Shining Armor and Bear Man.

Peter Tooker, my brother for his trustworthiness, quiet and gentle wisdom and brilliant sense of humor.

Sally Allison, my beautiful sister and best friend, compassionate and wise confidant, and loving giggle partner.

Michelle Vandepas, my amazing author and marketing coach with her Mastermind Matrix Leadership of Love.

Karen Curry Parker, my brilliant Human Design coach with her Mastermind Matrix Leadership of Compassion.

Camille Truman, my stellar book designer and publishing coordinator, who saw the Inner River of Peace and The Message Mandala flowing through the book.

Kimberly Leady, my patient graphic designer extraordinaire.

Life has a Way of its own: If I had not studied Brain Tracy's theories on Success in my real estate career, I would not have had a consultation with one of his coaches, David Nield. He led me to Michelle Vandepas and her tribe, and it all carried on from there. Divine timing and divine order are beautiful and amazing. Gratitude is in order.

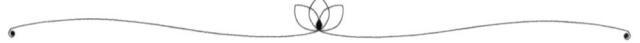

Honoring the Elders who reside in a precious place in my heart with their inspiration, wisdom, courage, compassion, and most of all their love.

Suzanne Whaley

Vera Lindabury

John R. Wood

David Melnik

The Late Madame Micheline Arcier

About the Author

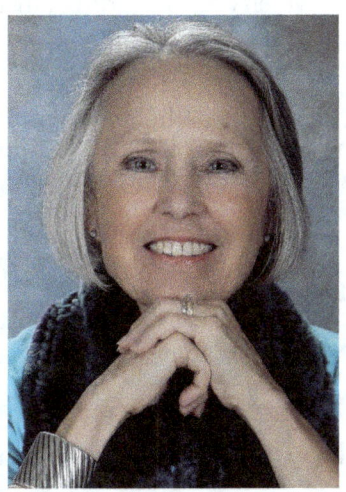

Candace Jean Newman MAT, LMT, The Oil Lady®, holds a Master of Arts in Teaching and is a Licensed Massage Therapist. Her work is based on the synergistic relationship of *Your Inner River of Peace: Ten Messages of Love*, the Ten Principles of Touch With Oils®, and the Touch With Oils® Hand Massage. These Motions in Stillness Methods create *The Circle of Compassion in Action* that encompasses this work.

Candace is one of the authors (referred to as *The Women of NAHA*) who wrote *The World of Aromatherapy*. She has written guides, educational newsletters, and numerous articles for national and international publications. Her courses and publications are available on her website.

The aromatherapy training and certificates Candace holds are from Purdue University and leading aromatherapists in the United States, Canada, England, France, and Germany. Candace is the founder of Oil Lady Aromatherapy® and The Good Medicine Tin®. She is the founder and owner of the Touch With Oils® Institute LLC. Touch With Oils® and The Oil Lady® are registered trademarks. All rights reserved.

www.TouchWithOilsInstitute.com

Other Publications by Candace:

Aromatherapy for Sleep

Aromatherapy for Stress

Aromatherapy for Anxiety

www.ingramcontent.com/pod-product-compliance
Lightning Source LLC
Chambersburg PA
CBHW071214080526
44587CB00013BA/1371